BY THE EDITORS OF CONSUMER GUIDE®

With Jeffrey W. Ellis, M.D.

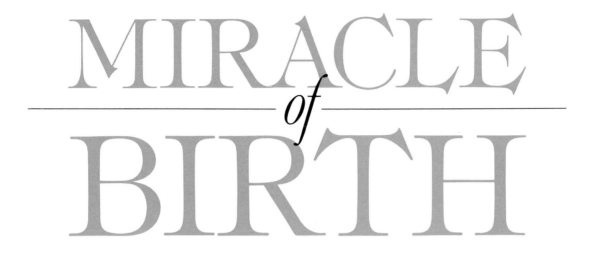

MIRACLE
*of*
BIRTH

Publications International, Ltd.

# CONTENTS

## THE FIRST TRIMESTER . . . . . . . . 8

### The First Month

### The Second Month

Common discomforts of the first trimester •
Psychological changes • Sexual relations •
Safeguarding your baby's health

### The Third Month

Louis Weber, C.E.O.
Publications International, Ltd.
7373 North Cicero Avenue
Lincolnwood, Illinois 60646

Printed in Yugoslavia, by Zrinski 1990.

h g f e d c b a

ISBN 0-88176-560-0

Library of Congress Catalog Card Number: 89-63240

# THE SECOND TRIMESTER ..... 44

**Author:** Jeffrey W. Ellis, M.D., is a board-certified obstetrician and gynecologist who took his M.D. degree at the University of Illinois. He is an assistant professor of health sciences and an associate professor of health care administration at Rosary College in River Forest, Illinois.
**Contributing author:** Marla Ellis, B.S.N., R.N., A.C.C.E.
**Anatomical illustrations:** Teri J. McDermott, M.A., Medical Illustrator and Sharon Kraus, M.A.M.S., Medical Illustrator. Copyright © 1989 McDermott/Kraus.
Front and back cover illustrations: Teri J. McDermott, M.A.
**Other illustrations:** Ilene Robinette.

# THE THIRD TRIMESTER ....... 78

## The Seventh Month

## The Eighth Month

## The Ninth Month

# LABOR AND DELIVERY ....... 108

# Introduction

Pregnancy and childbirth are supposed to be "natural" processes. So why do you have so many questions about what to do and what not to do now that you are pregnant?

Rest assured, you're experiencing what all first-time (and even many second- and third-time) mothers experience when they learn that they're pregnant. Pregnancy is a time of change and a time of choices, and it's natural to wonder what lies ahead.

In your grandmother's day, the process of carrying and delivering a child was governed by concern for the physical safety of the mother and baby. The choices concerning what to do and what not to do were limited.

Today, however, medical advances have made pregnancy and childbirth a great deal safer. Attention has now turned to making pregnancy a psychologically rewarding and more comfortable experience as well as a safe one.

With so many more options, it's not surprising that you have questions about pregnancy and childbirth. Nor is it surprising or abnormal for you to worry about yourself and your baby, regardless of the advances that modern medicine has wrought.

Fortunately, there are many things that you can do to help ensure your safety and the safety of your developing baby. There are also many ways to make childbirth a joyful and fulfilling experience.

Preparing for childbirth means eating properly, exercising, avoiding hazards, taking care of yourself, and learning all that you can about

---

## This book is designed to help you take good care of yourself and your baby during your pregnancy.

---

pregnancy, labor, and delivery. Even though you will see your doctor regularly throughout pregnancy, the best prenatal care is the care that you give yourself. Only you can make the daily commitment to a good diet, safe exercise and activity, and avoidance of harmful substances. Your doctor can only monitor your pregnancy, give you advice, and intervene if complications occur. You are ultimately responsible for caring for yourself and your developing baby.

That's where this book comes in. It's designed to answer your questions and give you the information you need to take good care of yourself and your baby during pregnancy. It will help you to understand and visualize how your baby develops, how your body changes, and how you can help ensure that your pregnancy and your baby are healthy. It also provides you with tips and suggestions for making pregnancy more comfortable and enjoyable.

Keep in mind that there isn't one specific way of doing things. Every pregnancy is unique, and therefore it is difficult to predict exactly what will occur and when. Only you and your doctor can decide what is best for you. What this book does is provide you with the information that you need so that you, your husband, and your doctor can make decisions together about your pregnancy, labor, and delivery.

**How This Book is Divided.** The information is divided into four major parts. The first three parts correspond to the three trimesters of your pregnancy. The final part covers labor and delivery.

Within each trimester, you will find the following sections:

- Your Growing Baby
- Your Changing Body
- Ask the Doctor
- For You and Your Baby
- Coping with the Changes
- Planning and Preparation
- Special Situations

The *Your Growing Baby* section appears three times in each trimester (once for every month in the trimester—nine times in all). This section discusses how your baby grows and develops during each month. It is here that you will discover when your baby's heart starts to beat and when his tiny fingers develop, as well as other details about his miraculous journey to birth.

The *Your Changing Body* section, which likewise appears three times in each trimester, describes and illustrates how your body changes in response to your growing baby. Here you will learn how your body adapts to pregnancy, how it nurtures your developing baby, and how it prepares for labor and delivery.

Each trimester also contains three monthly *Ask the Doctor* sections. Each of the *Doctor* sections covers a specific question that you may have about pregnancy, labor, or delivery, such as "How much weight should I gain?" and "How will I know if something is wrong?" At the end of each *Doctor* section, you will find a summary of what your doctor will probably do and what types of tests are usually performed during that month's prenatal doctor visit.

Within each trimester, you will also find a section called *For You and Your Baby*. This section deals with a specific aspect of prenatal care for you and your baby. In the first trimester, for example, *For You and Your Baby* covers proper nutrition during pregnancy; in the second trimester, safe exercise and activity; and in the third trimester, rest and relaxation.

Each trimester includes one *Coping with the Changes* section, which discusses the discomforts, both physical and psychological, that tend to occur in that trimester and what you can do to prevent or relieve them. The *Coping* sections also discuss sexual relations, safeguarding your developing baby's health, and dealing with

practical matters like choosing clothing and shoes for pregnancy.

The *Planning and Preparation* section occurs once in each trimester as well. Each *Planning* section deals with issues that you need to think about and discuss ahead of time. For example, in the first trimester, the *Planning* section discusses working and traveling throughout pregnancy. We talk about these issues in the

---

To prepare for the months ahead, read through the book early, then refer to specific months as you reach them.

---

first trimester because early in your pregnancy you will need to consult your doctor about how long you will be able to work and travel. Also, you will need to notify your employer as soon as possible about when you will need to take time off.

The final section in each trimester is called *Special Situations*. As the name implies, this section covers situations in pregnancy—such as carrying more than one baby—that may require a little extra attention, preparation, and caution.

After the three trimesters, you will find *Labor and Delivery*. This part of the book explains what labor is and gives you an idea of what's likely to happen during childbirth. We'll take you step by step through the childbirth process, from the moment you suspect you are in labor to that wondrous moment when your new baby is placed in your arms. You'll learn about the factors that influence labor and what you can do to help the process along. You'll find a handy chart that can help you distinguish between *real* labor and *false* labor. You'll also

find strategies for coping with the contractions that bring your baby closer to birth.

Within the book, you will also find a group of four full-color pages that illustrate, in vibrant detail, the wondrous changes that occur in your body and in your baby through the course of pregnancy. The first overlay illustrates early pregnancy; the tiny embryo is attached to the wall of the uterus and has begun the process of growth and development that will take him to full development. The second overlay shows the mother and the baby three months after conception. The third overlay illustrates the changes that occur by the end of the sixth month after conception. The final color page shows what the mother and fetus look like at term, when the baby has dropped lower in the abdomen in preparation for birth.

At the end of the book, you will find a handy glossary of the terms used throughout the book and a detailed index to help you locate the specific information you need quickly and easily.

**How to Use This Book.** While this book illustrates and describes the changes that occur in each month and each trimester of pregnancy, we encourage you to browse through the book early in pregnancy to get an idea of what's ahead and what types of preparations and precautions you can make to ensure a happy, healthy pregnancy and delivery. This is especially true for the *For You and Your Baby* sections, which cover important prenatal care topics like nutrition, exercise, and rest. Then, as you reach each specific month, you can turn to that section and explore, in detail, what's happening within your body.

We also encourage you to use the full-color overlays as a reference for other sections of the book. The fine detail and the clear labels will help you to visualize the changes occurring in your body and understand why you are experiencing the physical discomforts that occur during pregnancy.

As we've said, each pregnancy is unique. Not every pregnant woman experiences the exact same discomforts at the exact same time during pregnancy. Although most women experience "normal" or "typical" pregnancies, there is no strict definition of what that means. In addition, some women develop complications during

---

**We encourage you to refer to the four full-color illustrations as you read through the book.**

---

pregnancy that range from minor to severe.

In this book, we discuss the changes that typically occur and give you an idea of approximately when those changes are likely to take place. If you don't develop a symptom or change that is discussed here, it doesn't necessarily mean that something is wrong. Likewise, while we have tried to be thorough in our coverage of the changes and discomforts of pregnancy, you may develop a symptom that is not discussed here. Once again, that symptom may or may not signal a problem. Therefore, if you have any questions about what you're feeling—or what you aren't feeling—be sure to discuss them with your doctor.

As you read and refer to this book, you may notice that we refer to your relationship with your "husband" and the role that your "husband" may play during your pregnancy, labor, and delivery. We realize that there are a variety of circumstances under which pregnancy may occur and that not every woman goes through preg-

nancy, labor, and delivery with "her husband." We use this traditional term simply to avoid confusion, without meaning to imply that all women experience pregnancy and childbirth in the context of such a relationship.

You may also notice that we alternate, by trimester, our references to the gender of your baby and the gender of your doctor. This method was chosen in order to account for the obvious possibilities without making the references confusing.

This book is meant to give you the information and confidence you need to make pregnancy and childbirth a healthy, memorable,

and joyful time. We encourage you to refer to it often throughout your pregnancy and to use the information it contains to prepare yourself for the months ahead. By taking time now to learn about pregnancy and childbirth, you'll feel more at ease as you approach the birth of your child. You'll be better able to nurture yourself and your developing baby throughout pregnancy, and you'll be able to use the months of pregnancy to prepare your body and mind for labor and delivery. By beginning your preparations now, you'll have more energy to enjoy the miracle of birth and to savor that first moment, when you hold your beautiful new baby in your arms.

---

## A Note About How Pregnancy is Calculated

We chose to divide this book into trimesters because pregnancy has traditionally been referred to in terms of three trimesters, each lasting approximately three months. The first trimester of a woman's pregnancy is considered to begin on the first day of her last menstrual period, and it is from this date that the estimated date of delivery is calculated.

Now, you may be saying to yourself, "Wait a minute. How could I have gotten pregnant on the first day of my last menstrual period?" Indeed, you may even be able to pinpoint the exact day that you did conceive.

For many women, however, it is difficult to pinpoint the day that conception occurred. Although ovulation usually occurs about two weeks after the start of the menstrual cycle, not every woman's cycle is the same. So to simplify matters, a woman's pregnancy has traditionally been referred to as beginning on the first day of her last normal menstrual period, even though she may have conceived one, two, or even three weeks after that date. To put it another way, when you've reached the end of your

calculated first month of pregnancy, your baby may actually be only one, two, or three weeks old.

The illustrations and text throughout this book take into account the difference between when *tradition* says your pregnancy began and when you actually conceived. For example, when we discuss the changes that occur in the woman's body during the first month, we are referring to the *traditional* first month of pregnancy, which begins on the first day of the last menstrual period. When we discuss how the baby changes in the first month, however, we are referring to the actual first month of pregnancy, which began at conception. (The monthly illustrations of mother and baby, as well as the full-color overlays, show the changes in terms of the age of the developing baby.)

There's no need to be concerned about this distinction. After all, each pregnancy is unique, and the changes do not happen at exactly the same time in each woman. The descriptions and illustrations are designed to give you a general idea of how your baby and your body change as pregnancy progresses.

# THE
# FIRST
# TRIMESTER

**D**iscovering that you are pregnant is an exciting moment. It is the start of a period of wonder and waiting, anticipation and expectation, and above all, change.

In the first three months of your pregnancy—known as your first trimester—you will begin to notice physical as well as emotional changes. The physical changes may, at times, be uncomfortable. The emotional changes may confuse or even frighten you. But rest assured that, in most instances, these changes are normal. They are necessary changes that prepare your body and your mind to nurture the baby that is developing within you.

Indeed, within three months after conception, every organ that your baby will need throughout her life will have formed. Some, such as her tiny heart and kidneys, will have already begun to function. Because your first trimester of pregnancy is such a critical period in your baby's development, you need to take extra-special care of yourself during this time.

In the following sections, we'll describe how your baby develops during her first three months in the womb, and we'll discuss the changes that will occur in your body. To help you nurture yourself and provide your baby with all that she needs during this time of rapid development, you'll find information on proper diet, weight gain, prenatal doctor visits, and working during pregnancy. You'll also find helpful tips to decrease the discomforts that can accompany the many changes taking place.

# Your Growing Baby

Conception occurs when an egg from your ovary is fertilized by a single sperm. This process usually takes place about two weeks after the start of your last menstrual period. The result of this union of an egg and a sperm is a single cell—the beginning of your baby. Even at this earliest stage of development, all of your baby's characteristics—sex, hair color, eye color, blood type, and so on—have been determined.

The egg and sperm unite within the fallopian tube, the four-inch long passageway that connects the ovary to the uterus. Within hours, the fertilized egg begins to divide and slowly floats toward the cavity of the uterus. In a matter of days, the fertilized egg—which is now a tightly packed cluster of many cells—fastens itself to the wall of the uterus to obtain nutrients and shelter. It is within the uterus that your baby grows and develops during pregnancy.

Once implanted in the wall of the uterus, this tiny mass of cells, now called an embryo, begins dividing into new cells that will eventually form all of the organs of your baby's body. Each of these new cells is unique; each has a special mission. Some of the new cells go on to form your baby's heart, while others are destined to form her brain, liver, kidneys, stomach, and other organs.

As these first cells continue to increase in size and number, great changes take place. Some of these cells begin to burrow into the wall of your uterus to form the placenta. This amazing organ—also called the afterbirth—will soon be attached to your baby via the umbilical cord and will provide a vital link through which oxygen and nutrients from your body are transferred to your baby. (Before the fertilized egg implants in the uterine wall, the baby's cells obtain most of their nourishment from the fluids within the fallopian tube. After implantation, a balloonlike structure called the yolk sac forms to supply nourishment to the developing embryo until the placenta is developed enough to take over this role.)

Within a few more days, a tiny water-tight sac—called the amniotic sac or "bag of waters"—forms around your developing baby and gradually fills with clear fluid. This amniotic sac cushions the growing baby from shocks while at the same time allowing her to move around freely—raising her arms and even doing flips.

One month after conception, the original fertilized egg has undergone many dramatic changes. Your growing baby is now nearly 10,000 times larger than the single cell from which she came. Her tiny developing body has a head, as well as small buds that will become her arms and legs. Though she is only about a quarter of an inch long, her face is beginning to form and tiny dark circles appear where her eyes will be. Her mouth, lower jaw, and throat also begin to develop.

Internally, your baby is starting to develop organs that, in the next few months, will grow and eventually begin to function. During the first month of development, cells in different parts of the baby's body begin to form her lungs, kidneys, liver, and brain. A small tube that will become the baby's heart forms, and by the end of the month, it actually starts beating, although far too faintly to be heard by you or your doctor.

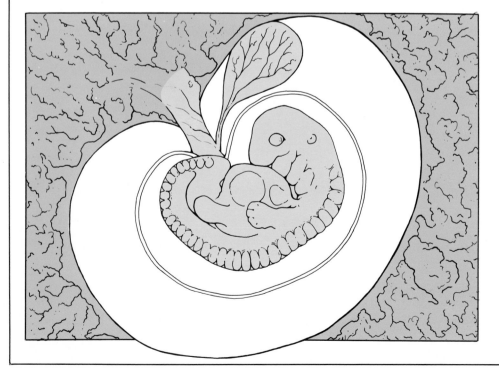

# MONTH

# Your Changing Body

Perhaps the first thing you will notice when you are pregnant is that you have missed your menstrual period. During a normal menstrual cycle, the hormones estrogen and progesterone, which are produced by your ovaries, cause a buildup of tissue and blood vessels in the inner walls of your uterus. This is the body's way of preparing for the fertilized egg if you should become pregnant. If your egg is not fertilized by a sperm, the thickened lining of your uterus is sloughed away at the end of the month and you have a menstrual period. If your egg is fertilized, however, the lining of the uterus does not slough away. Instead, it grows even thicker and forms the attachment for the placenta (the organ that develops on the inner wall of the uterus to supply nutrients to your baby and carry the baby's waste products back to your body to be excreted).

While you are pregnant, you will not have periods. During the first month of pregnancy, however, some women will notice very slight bleeding or light brown vaginal discharge at the time of the month when their period would usually occur. This is quite normal and is thought to be a result of the implanting of the placenta in the inner wall of the uterus. If you notice any bleeding after the first month, however, you should report it to your doctor immediately.

When you visit your doctor for the first time during your pregnancy, you will be asked for the date that your last *normal* menstrual period began. This date is used to calculate the due date for your pregnancy. If possible, keep careful track of the dates of your last normal menstrual period and any other episodes of bleeding or spotting. This will help eliminate errors in calculating your due date (see page 12 for more on calculating your due date).

Another sign that may indicate that you are pregnant is the sudden onset of nausea and vomiting—commonly called morning sickness. About two-thirds of all pregnant women experience this type of

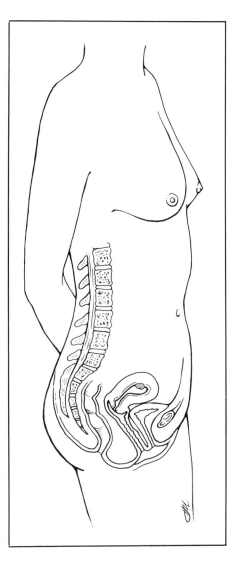

discomfort. It commonly occurs in the morning (hence its name) but may also develop at any time of the day. Morning sickness may be

---

## Keep careful track of the dates of your last period.

---

triggered by a hormone called human chorionic gonadotropin, which is produced by the placenta; however, emotional factors and even unpleasant odors may also play a role. Fortunately, morning sickness is usually easy to control (see *Coping*, page 27) and generally does not last beyond the first trimester. If you experience severe morning sickness, however, your doctor may have you modify your diet or may prescribe medication to relieve the nausea and vomiting.

Another change that you are likely to notice is the need to urinate more frequently, sometimes even during the middle of the night. When you are not pregnant, your uterus lies wholly within the bony cavity of the pelvis. The bladder, which stores your urine, lies in front of the uterus, also within the pelvic cavity. As your uterus enlarges during the first trimester, it pushes against the bladder and decreases the bladder's capacity to hold urine. As a result, you will urinate more frequently and usually in smaller amounts. During the second trimester, the uterus grows upward into the abdominal cavity, relieving the pressure on your bladder and allowing you to urinate less frequently.

# What Happens at the First Prenatal Visit?

Since the well-being of your baby will depend on your health during pregnancy, it is always best to place yourself under the care of a doctor as soon as possible.

Your first prenatal appointment with your doctor should occur as soon as you think you are pregnant, usually about two weeks after you miss your menstrual period. Since the well-being of your baby will depend on your health during pregnancy, it is always best to place yourself under the care of a doctor as soon as possible.

During the first visit, your doctor will take a thorough medical history and will perform a complete physical examination. Certain laboratory tests will also be performed to detect any abnormalities in your blood, urine, and reproductive organs.

You will also have an opportunity to discuss with your doctor any questions and concerns that you have about your pregnancy. It's a good idea to jot these down before you actually visit the doctor.

To help you prepare, here's a summary of the types of questions, procedures, and tests that are generally part of the first prenatal visit.

**Current Symptoms.** The first question that your doctor will ask you is "When was your last normal menstrual period?" Since this information is very important for calculating your expected delivery date ("due date") and for performing certain tests on you and the baby, you should bring an accurate record of the dates of your periods. Also, you should note any other spotting or unusual bleeding and report it to your doctor.

Your doctor will ask you about other symptoms of pregnancy—such as morning sickness, breast tenderness, and frequent urination—that you may be experiencing. He may also ask you about other symptoms—such as a sore throat or coughing—that may indicate illness.

**Calculating Your Delivery Date.** Once he has determined the dates of your last menstrual period, your doctor will be able to calculate your expected date of delivery and tell you how far along you are in your pregnancy.

The average length of pregnancy is 280 days from the first day of the last normal menstrual period. Of course, conception may actually occur one, two, or three weeks after the start of the last period. But since it is difficult to pinpoint exactly when conception occurs, the first date of the last menstrual period has traditionally been used as the starting point for calculating the length of pregnancy and the estimated delivery date.

One way to determine your due date is to count 280 days forward from the first day of your last menstrual period.

A simpler way to calculate your due date is to add nine months and seven days to the first day of your last menstrual period. For example, if your last menstrual period began on January 10, adding nine months and seven days would give you a due date of October 17. Still another way to determine your due date is to use the chart on page 13.

Very few women actually deliver their babies exactly on their due date. Usually, it's a few days before or a few days after. However, nearly 95 percent of babies are delivered within two weeks of their calculated delivery date.

**Your Medical History.** Next, your doctor will ask you questions about current illnesses, previous illnesses, and previous pregnancies. Certain illnesses and problems in the mother may cause complications during pregnancy, so your doctor may need to perform special tests or examine you more frequently if you have any such

# Estimated Date of Delivery

| LMP = Jan. | 1 | 2 | 3 | 4 | 5 | 6 | 7 | 8 | 9 | 10 | 11 | 12 | 13 | 14 | 15 | 16 | 17 | 18 | 19 | 20 | 21 | 22 | 23 | 24 | 25 | 26 | 27 | 28 | 29 | 30 | 31 | Jan. |
|---|---|---|---|---|---|---|---|---|---|---|---|---|---|---|---|---|---|---|---|---|---|---|---|---|---|---|---|---|---|---|---|---|
| EDD = Oct. | 8 | 9 | 10 | 11 | 12 | 13 | 14 | 15 | 16 | 17 | 18 | 19 | 20 | 21 | 22 | 23 | 24 | 25 | 26 | 27 | 28 | 29 | 30 | 31 | 1 | 2 | 3 | 4 | 5 | 6 | 7 | Nov. |
| LMP = Feb. | 1 | 2 | 3 | 4 | 5 | 6 | 7 | 8 | 9 | 10 | 11 | 12 | 13 | 14 | 15 | 16 | 17 | 18 | 19 | 20 | 21 | 22 | 23 | 24 | 25 | 26 | 27 | 28 | | | | Feb. |
| EDD = Nov. | 8 | 9 | 10 | 11 | 12 | 13 | 14 | 15 | 16 | 17 | 18 | 19 | 20 | 21 | 22 | 23 | 24 | 25 | 26 | 27 | 28 | 29 | 30 | 1 | 2 | 3 | 4 | 5 | | | | Dec. |
| LMP = Mar. | 1 | 2 | 3 | 4 | 5 | 6 | 7 | 8 | 9 | 10 | 11 | 12 | 13 | 14 | 15 | 16 | 17 | 18 | 19 | 20 | 21 | 22 | 23 | 24 | 25 | 26 | 27 | 28 | 29 | 30 | 31 | Mar. |
| EDD = Dec. | 6 | 7 | 8 | 9 | 10 | 11 | 12 | 13 | 14 | 15 | 16 | 17 | 18 | 19 | 20 | 21 | 22 | 23 | 24 | 25 | 26 | 27 | 28 | 29 | 30 | 31 | 1 | 2 | 3 | 4 | 5 | Jan. |
| LMP = April | 1 | 2 | 3 | 4 | 5 | 6 | 7 | 8 | 9 | 10 | 11 | 12 | 13 | 14 | 15 | 16 | 17 | 18 | 19 | 20 | 21 | 22 | 23 | 24 | 25 | 26 | 27 | 28 | 29 | 30 | | April |
| EDD = Jan. | 6 | 7 | 8 | 9 | 10 | 11 | 12 | 13 | 14 | 15 | 16 | 17 | 18 | 19 | 20 | 21 | 22 | 23 | 24 | 25 | 26 | 27 | 28 | 29 | 30 | 31 | 1 | 2 | 3 | 4 | | Feb. |
| LMP = May | 1 | 2 | 3 | 4 | 5 | 6 | 7 | 8 | 9 | 10 | 11 | 12 | 13 | 14 | 15 | 16 | 17 | 18 | 19 | 20 | 21 | 22 | 23 | 24 | 25 | 26 | 27 | 28 | 29 | 30 | 31 | May |
| EDD = Feb. | 5 | 6 | 7 | 8 | 9 | 10 | 11 | 12 | 13 | 14 | 15 | 16 | 17 | 18 | 19 | 20 | 21 | 22 | 23 | 24 | 25 | 26 | 27 | 28 | 1 | 2 | 3 | 4 | 5 | 6 | 7 | Mar. |
| LMP = June | 1 | 2 | 3 | 4 | 5 | 6 | 7 | 8 | 9 | 10 | 11 | 12 | 13 | 14 | 15 | 16 | 17 | 18 | 19 | 20 | 21 | 22 | 23 | 24 | 25 | 26 | 27 | 28 | 29 | 30 | | June |
| EDD = Mar. | 8 | 9 | 10 | 11 | 12 | 13 | 14 | 15 | 16 | 17 | 18 | 19 | 20 | 21 | 22 | 23 | 24 | 25 | 26 | 27 | 28 | 29 | 30 | 31 | 1 | 2 | 3 | 4 | 5 | 6 | | April |
| LMP = July | 1 | 2 | 3 | 4 | 5 | 6 | 7 | 8 | 9 | 10 | 11 | 12 | 13 | 14 | 15 | 16 | 17 | 18 | 19 | 20 | 21 | 22 | 23 | 24 | 25 | 26 | 27 | 28 | 29 | 30 | 31 | July |
| EDD = April | 7 | 8 | 9 | 10 | 11 | 12 | 13 | 14 | 15 | 16 | 17 | 18 | 19 | 20 | 21 | 22 | 23 | 24 | 25 | 26 | 27 | 28 | 29 | 30 | 1 | 2 | 3 | 4 | 5 | 6 | 7 | May |
| LMP = Aug. | 1 | 2 | 3 | 4 | 5 | 6 | 7 | 8 | 9 | 10 | 11 | 12 | 13 | 14 | 15 | 16 | 17 | 18 | 19 | 20 | 21 | 22 | 23 | 24 | 25 | 26 | 27 | 28 | 29 | 30 | 31 | Aug. |
| EDD = May | 8 | 9 | 10 | 11 | 12 | 13 | 14 | 15 | 16 | 17 | 18 | 19 | 20 | 21 | 22 | 23 | 24 | 25 | 26 | 27 | 28 | 29 | 30 | 31 | 1 | 2 | 3 | 4 | 5 | 6 | 7 | June |
| LMP = Sept. | 1 | 2 | 3 | 4 | 5 | 6 | 7 | 8 | 9 | 10 | 11 | 12 | 13 | 14 | 15 | 16 | 17 | 18 | 19 | 20 | 21 | 22 | 23 | 24 | 25 | 26 | 27 | 28 | 29 | 30 | | Sept. |
| EDD = June | 8 | 9 | 10 | 11 | 12 | 13 | 14 | 15 | 16 | 17 | 18 | 19 | 20 | 21 | 22 | 23 | 24 | 25 | 26 | 27 | 28 | 29 | 30 | 1 | 2 | 3 | 4 | 5 | 6 | 7 | | July |
| LMP = Oct. | 1 | 2 | 3 | 4 | 5 | 6 | 7 | 8 | 9 | 10 | 11 | 12 | 13 | 14 | 15 | 16 | 17 | 18 | 19 | 20 | 21 | 22 | 23 | 24 | 25 | 26 | 27 | 28 | 29 | 30 | 31 | Oct. |
| EDD = July | 8 | 9 | 10 | 11 | 12 | 13 | 14 | 15 | 16 | 17 | 18 | 19 | 20 | 21 | 22 | 23 | 24 | 25 | 26 | 27 | 28 | 29 | 30 | 31 | 1 | 2 | 3 | 4 | 5 | 6 | 7 | Aug. |
| LMP = Nov. | 1 | 2 | 3 | 4 | 5 | 6 | 7 | 8 | 9 | 10 | 11 | 12 | 13 | 14 | 15 | 16 | 17 | 18 | 19 | 20 | 21 | 22 | 23 | 24 | 25 | 26 | 27 | 28 | 29 | 30 | | Nov. |
| EDD = Aug. | 8 | 9 | 10 | 11 | 12 | 13 | 14 | 15 | 16 | 17 | 18 | 19 | 20 | 21 | 22 | 23 | 24 | 25 | 26 | 27 | 28 | 29 | 30 | 31 | 1 | 2 | 3 | 4 | 5 | 6 | | Sept. |
| LMP = Dec. | 1 | 2 | 3 | 4 | 5 | 6 | 7 | 8 | 9 | 10 | 11 | 12 | 13 | 14 | 15 | 16 | 17 | 18 | 19 | 20 | 21 | 22 | 23 | 24 | 25 | 26 | 27 | 28 | 29 | 30 | 31 | Dec. |
| EDD = Sept. | 7 | 8 | 9 | 10 | 11 | 12 | 13 | 14 | 15 | 16 | 17 | 18 | 19 | 20 | 21 | 22 | 23 | 24 | 25 | 26 | 27 | 28 | 29 | 30 | 1 | 2 | 3 | 4 | 5 | 6 | 7 | Oct. |

To find the estimated date of your baby's birth, find the black date that corresponds to the first day of your last menstrual period (LMP). The colored number just below it is your estimated date of delivery (EDD).

illness. Among the illnesses that may complicate pregnancy are heart disease, kidney disease, diabetes, high blood pressure, and certain infections.

Complications that occurred in a previous pregnancy may also repeat themselves in your current pregnancy. For this reason, your doctor will ask you many detailed questions about any previous pregnancies or miscarriages. Your answers will help your doctor to anticipate complications and either prevent them or treat them early. The information that your doctor will need concerning any previous pregnancies includes:

- Date of delivery
- Length of pregnancy
- Length of labor
- Complications, if any, that arose in pregnancy, labor, delivery, or postpartum (after delivery)
- Type of delivery (spontaneous, forceps, or cesarean section)
- Condition of the baby at birth

If you had any complications with a previous pregnancy and you are now seeing a different doctor, try to obtain your previous medical records and bring them with you to the first visit.

Your doctor will also ask you about any medications that you are currently taking. In some cases, he may ask you to stop taking them if there is any chance that they may be harmful to the baby. If you are unsure of what medications you are taking, bring the prescription containers with you.

**Family History.** During your first visit, your doctor will inquire about the health of your husband, brothers, sisters, parents, and other close family members. The purpose is to determine if there are any illnesses that may first become apparent during your pregnancy. Diabetes and high blood pressure, for example, tend to run in families and may first produce symptoms in a woman during the stressful period of pregnancy.

Your doctor will also want to know if any family members have birth defects or other illnesses that may be inherited by your baby.

**Social History.** Your doctor will ask you questions about your social history, including your occupation, your physical activities and hobbies, and your habits, such as cigarette smoking and use of alcohol or drugs. These questions should always be answered honestly, since the purpose is to determine if the baby will be exposed to any harmful substances or physical injury. Your doctor will counsel you to stop certain activities or discontinue the use of certain substances if they are potentially hazardous to your pregnancy.

**Physical Examination.** After the doctor has completed taking your medical history, you will be asked to undress and put on a gown. Your doctor will then give you a complete physical examination. Usually, a nurse will have determined your height, weight, and blood pressure before the doctor begins. The doctor will carefully and systematically check your eyes, mouth, chest, heartbeat, breasts, abdomen, and legs for the presence of any abnormality that may indicate illness or complicate pregnancy.

Next, your doctor will perform a pelvic examination to determine the size of your uterus and to detect any abnormality of the ovaries, fallopian tubes, cervix, vagina, or external sexual organs. He will also carefully feel the bones of your pelvis to determine if the pelvis is large enough for a safe delivery.

At this time, the doctor will also take a Pap smear from your cervix to detect any cancerous cells and may perform cultures to detect any infections of the cervix or vagina that may affect the baby.

If it has been more than 12 weeks since the start of your last menstrual period, your doctor will also listen for the baby's heartbeat using a microphonelike instrument called a doppler. If you are past the fifth month, he may be able to hear the heartbeat with a stethoscope.

After the first visit, the doctor will not need to repeat a complete physical examination. However, at each subsequent visit, he will check your weight and blood pressure, measure the size of your uterus, listen to the baby's heartbeat, and, toward the end of pregnancy, check the position of the baby. He may also examine other parts of your body if you are experiencing discomfort, such as soreness of the legs or headache.

**Blood and Urine Tests.** During your first visit, your doctor will also order certain tests to be performed on your urine and blood. The nurse will generally ask you to urinate into a small cup before you undress for the physical examination. Some doctors may instead ask that you obtain your urine sample at home and bring it with you to your appointment.

Your urine will be checked for the presence of sugar (glucose) and protein (albumin). The presence of sugar in the urine may indicate that you have diabetes; the presence of protein may indicate kidney disease. If you have either of these conditions during pregnancy, it is important that they be diagnosed. A small portion of the urine sample may also be sent to a laboratory to check for signs of kidney or bladder infection.

If you are early in your pregnancy, the nurse will usually perform a pregnancy test on your urine. If, however, you are quite advanced in your pregnancy, with an obviously protruding abdomen, the pregnancy test will not be necessary.

Several small tubes of your blood will also be drawn by either the nurse or a laboratory technician. The samples of your blood will be sent to a laboratory to determine your blood type, Rh factor (see page 70), glucose (sugar) level, blood cell count, and immunity to German measles (Rubella). If your blood does not indicate that you are immune to German measles, you will be advised to avoid contact with anyone who has this disease.

Your blood may also be tested for the presence of syphilis, AIDS, and other sexually transmitted diseases. If you have a personal or family history of certain illnesses,

additional blood tests may also be performed.

Some of these tests will be repeated during future office visits. During each visit, the nurse will check your urine for sugar and protein. During the fifth month of pregnancy, another blood test will be done to check your blood sugar level. Your blood count will usually be checked again during the eighth month.

**Counseling.** After you dress, the doctor will sit down with you and offer practical advice for the early stages of pregnancy, discuss any abnormal findings, and answer any of your questions. At this time, it is also best to discuss any plans that you have made regarding childbirth education classes, use of anesthesia during labor (see page 90), breast-feeding, and so on.

During this discussion, the doctor will also talk about your diet, weight gain, physical activity, clothing, and hygiene. He will describe to you the "warning signs" of pregnancy that may indicate that a complication is developing. Be sure to get the doctor's emergency telephone numbers and the telephone number of the hospital just in case you need to reach him when he is not in the office.

Your doctor will also tell you when you should return for future visits. Generally, during the first 28 weeks of your pregnancy, you will be seen by the doctor once a month; from weeks 29 to 36, you will be seen once every two weeks; and from 36 weeks until delivery, you will be seen once a week. If you become ill or if complications develop, your doctor will examine you more frequently.

**Medications.** Before you leave his office, the doctor will usually write you prescriptions for an iron tablet and a multivitamin that is made specifically for pregnant women. Because the baby makes many nutritional demands on your body, you will normally need these supplements to your diet. Be sure that you take them as directed.

## This Month's Visit

During this month's office visit, the doctor will probably:

- Ask about symptoms of pregnancy. By now, you will have missed a menstrual period and may have morning sickness, breast tenderness, and a need to urinate more frequently.
- Calculate your expected date of delivery. The doctor will need to know the first day of your last normal menstrual period.
- Take a complete medical history and ask about current illnesses, previous illnesses, and previous pregnancies.
- Take a complete family history and ask about illnesses or birth defects in your husband, brothers, sisters, parents, and other close family members.
- Take a complete social history and ask about your occupation, physical activity, hobbies, and use of cigarettes, alcohol, and drugs.
- Check your height, weight, and blood pressure.
- Perform a complete physical examination.
- Perform a pelvic examination.
- Perform a Pap smear and take cultures from the vagina and cervix.
- Perform a pregnancy test, if necessary.
- Take blood samples to test for your blood type, Rh factor, blood count, sugar level, and immunity to German measles.
- Take blood samples to test for syphilis and AIDS.
- Give advice about symptoms of pregnancy.
- Discuss diet, weight gain, activity, clothing, and hygiene.
- Describe the danger signs of pregnancy.
- Prescribe multivitamins and iron tablets.

# Nutrition for a Healthy Pregnancy

The attention you give to good nutrition during pregnancy can greatly influence your baby's health as well as your own. Your diet during your pregnancy provides the essential building blocks for your developing baby's growth. You will want to consume the most nutritious foods to help build your baby's heart, lungs, brain, and skeleton. Eating well during pregnancy is a gift to your baby for life. It's also a way of nurturing yourself. Eating well makes you feel good, and it contributes to a healthy pregnancy.

Ideally, nutrition for pregnancy begins before conception, as you build up your stores of iron, calcium, and other nutrients. But it is never too late to pay attention to what you eat. You will feel better and your baby will benefit from the healthy changes in your diet.

In years past, nutrition advice to pregnant women differed greatly from what you will be told today. Weight gain was severely limited; salt was eliminated from the diet; and diuretics (drugs to stimulate urine production), laxatives, and even diet pills were routinely prescribed. Today, however, we know the importance of good nutrition and adequate weight gain during pregnancy for producing a full-term, vigorous infant and for contributing to a healthy pregnancy.

So read on, and discover how relatively simple it can be to provide you and your baby with the nutrients you both need by choosing foods wisely. And remember that if you have any questions about your diet or about specific foods, consult your doctor.

**How Much Should I Eat?** It's often said that a pregnant woman must eat for two. Unfortunately, many people believe that means that a pregnant woman must greatly increase the amount of food she eats. But that simply isn't true. While gaining enough weight is important, you need to realize that the other person you're eating for is a tiny developing person who doesn't require as much food as an adult—or even as much as a child. Indeed, the amount of food consumed by a pregnant woman is only slightly more than she is accustomed to eating when not pregnant—about 300 calories more per day.

The best way to interpret "eating for two" is to remember that when you feed yourself, you're also feeding your baby. If you make poor food choices for yourself, you're making the same ones for your baby. On the other hand, if you choose healthy, nutritious foods, you'll be providing your baby with the nutrients she needs for healthy development.

The recommended daily caloric intake during pregnancy is 2,100 to 2,400 calories. Your weight gain is a good guide to how well you are meeting your caloric requirements (see *Ask the Doctor*, page 24, for more on weight gain).

When fulfilling your daily energy needs, you'll want to choose foods that provide not only calories but vitamins, minerals, and other nutrients. Your requirements for certain nutrients increase in pregnancy, so you'll want to pay special attention to these.

**Protein.** Protein is essential for the development and maintenance of your baby's cells and organs. You need it, too, not only for normal cell growth and repair, but also for normal growth of the uterus, placenta, and breasts. Recommended daily amounts of protein increase dramatically from 46 grams (g) a day before pregnancy to 76 grams a day during pregnancy.

Since a deficiency of protein in the mother's diet has been associated with growth-retarded babies, it is very important that you always include sufficient amounts of protein in your diet. Good sources of protein are meat, poultry, fish, cheese, eggs, grains, nuts, milk, and legumes. Be sure to include them in your daily diet.

**Iron.** There are three major reasons for getting enough iron during pregnancy. First, iron is necessary for the formation of the mother's and the baby's hemoglobin, the oxygen-carrying component of blood. Since your blood volume increases considerably during pregnancy, and since your baby is also manufacturing her own blood cells, your need for iron increases. Second, during the last trimester, the baby draws iron from your body to store in her liver for use after she is born. Third, your increased blood volume and iron stores help your body adjust to the blood loss that occurs during childbirth.

Chances are, your doctor prescribed an iron supplement for you at your first prenatal visit. It's estimated that a pregnant woman needs just over 18 milligrams (mg) of iron each day. You may wonder, therefore, why your prenatal vitamin contains 30 to 60 milligrams of iron. This is because your stomach and intestines cannot totally absorb iron from supplements. So, you must ingest about 60 milligrams of iron to ensure that you actually absorb the required amount.

Iron supplements are best absorbed when they are taken with foods that are rich in vitamin C, such as orange juice, grapefruit, and strawberries. Absorption is slowed down if you take iron supplements with an antacid.

Some iron supplements may sometimes cause stomach upset, constipation, or nausea. If this is the case with you, your doctor may be able to prescribe another iron supplement that has fewer side effects.

Even though you may be taking iron supplements, it is still important that you eat foods rich in iron. These foods include liver, red meat, egg yolk, and legumes.

**Calcium.** Your calcium needs increase during pregnancy from 800 to 1,200 milligrams a day. Calcium is essential for the development and growth of your baby's skeleton, heart, muscles, and tooth buds. Inadequate calcium intake results in your own stores of calcium being depleted.

Milk and milk products (such as yogurt and cheese) are the best sources of dietary calcium. If you are intolerant of milk, as many adults are, your doctor may prescribe a calcium supplement for you.

**Vitamins.** The recommended daily allowances of nearly all vitamins increase in pregnancy by about 25 to 50 percent. Though your doctor will usually prescribe a vitamin supplement, it is still important for you to get adequate amounts of certain vitamins through your diet. All vitamins are important for your health, but the following are especially important in pregnancy.

*Folic Acid.* The recommended daily allowance for folic acid doubles during pregnancy from 400 micrograms (mcg) to 800 micrograms. Too little folic acid can cause a form of anemia in the pregnant woman that is characterized by the formation of abnormal red blood cells.

Although a high-quality, varied diet will supply most of the vitamins you will need for a healthy pregnancy, it may not provide you with enough folic acid. Therefore, supplements that provide 200 to 400 micrograms of folic acid are recommended in order to ensure that you are getting enough of this vitamin.

Since adequate folic acid intake is so important, you also need to adopt a diet that is rich in foods containing this essential vitamin. Liver, lean beef, legumes, egg yolks, and leafy, dark-green vegetables are good food sources of folic acid.

*Vitamin C.* This vitamin is essential for growth and maintenance of body tissues, resistance to infection, healing, and maintenance of bones and muscle. It also plays a key role in the absorption of iron.

The recommended daily allowance during pregnancy is 60 milligrams; during lactation, it rises to 80 milligrams. Sources of vitamin C are citrus fruits, tomatoes, potatoes, and leafy, green vegetables.

*Vitamin D.* Vitamin D is essential for the proper absorption of calcium and phosphorus in your body. It is also vital to the formation of healthy bones and teeth in your developing baby.

During pregnancy, a woman needs 400 International Units (IU) of vitamin D daily. Vitamin D can be acquired either through foods or through exposure to sunlight (your skin can manufacture vitamin D when you are exposed to the sun's ultraviolet light). Good food sources of vitamin D are fortified milk, margarine, fish, egg yolks, and yeast.

*Vitamin A.* The pregnant woman needs this vitamin for the maintenance of healthy skin and hair and for the proper functioning of her thyroid gland (the organ in the neck that secretes hormones that regulate metabolism). In the baby, vitamin A is necessary for bone growth and the development of tooth buds.

Foods containing vitamin A include butter, fortified margarine, cream, dark-green and deep-yellow vegetables, liver, and yellow noncitrus fruits.

**General Guidelines.** Dividing foods into specific food groups and then choosing servings from each group is a good way to be sure that you are getting the variety and quantity of nutrients you need for a healthy pregnancy. While you may be familiar with the "Basic Four" food groups plan, this breakdown may not be adequate to ensure that you get all the nutrients you need. Instead, you can divide foods into the following seven food categories and three nonfood categories.

- Dairy
- High-quality protein
- Grains and breads
- Green and yellow vegetables
- Citrus fruits; fruits and vegetables rich in vitamin C
- Potatoes and other vegetables and fruits
- Fats
- Fluids
- Iodine-containing foods
- Foods consisting primarily of nonnutritious calories

You can use the "Daily Food Guide" chart on pages 20–21 to record your daily diet and assess where changes need to be made. The chart lists each food group, tells you why it's important, specifies the number of servings

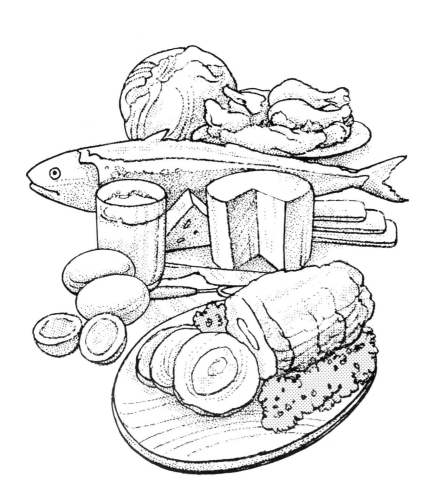

needed daily, and gives you examples of single servings. You'll find a space to record the number of servings you actually get each day. And, for the days when you don't get the required number of servings, you'll find a space to jot down the number of additional servings that you should have consumed to fulfill your requirements.

Keep track of your intake for several days, and then use the chart to analyze your diet. Are you neglecting certain food groups? Are you not getting enough of certain kinds of foods?

At first glance, the recommended numbers of servings may seem like too much food. However, on checking the size of the sample portions, you will find that the amount of food recommended is not at all excessive.

Sometimes your capacity or appetite is diminished, especially during late pregnancy or if you are experiencing heartburn or nausea. Eating several small meals during the day instead of three large meals may help to alleviate this problem.

Let your weight be your guide for how much food to eat. Your doctor will weigh you at each office visit to make sure that you are not gaining too little or too much. Any concerns you have about the amount of food you need should be shared with your doctor.

Some doctors will prescribe prenatal vitamins, while others may prescribe only folic acid supplements or iron supplements. Remember that these supplements are not a substitute for good food. They supply only some of the nutrients needed for health. The

rest you must get from the nutritious food that you eat.

**Vegetarian Diets.** If you are a vegetarian, you may need a little extra help in planning your diet during pregnancy. The following general guidelines will help, but if you have additional questions, be sure to discuss them with a doctor or dietician.

- Weight gain is a good indicator of adequate caloric intake.
- If you do not eat dairy products, you may need vitamin $B_{12}$, vitamin D, and calcium supplements.
- Pay special attention to getting enough protein by making meals with complementary proteins.
- Let your doctor know you are vegetarian.

**Teenage Pregnancy.** An adolescent mother-to-be needs special guidance during pregnancy because her diet must supply nutrients and calories to meet her own growth needs as well as those of her baby. The increased incidence of preeclampsia (a serious condition involving very high blood pressure) in pregnant teenagers may be related to an inadequate diet. Pregnant teenagers, therefore, need individualized nutritional counseling that is aimed at meeting their nutritional requirements.

**Multiple Pregnancy.** If you are carrying more than one baby, you will need to consume more calories and nutrients than you would if you were carrying only one child. If you are expecting two babies, for example, your requirement for iron will be double the requirement for a single pregnancy, so your doctor will need to increase your iron supplement. Your doctor will also advise you on how to appropriately increase your food intake.

**Foods to Avoid.** A variety of changes in the digestive system occur during pregnancy as a result of your changing hormone levels and the pressure of your enlarging uterus. For this reason, you may no longer be able to tolerate certain foods that you enjoyed before pregnancy. For example, gas pain is a common problem during pregnancy, since the entire digestive system slows down in response to the hormone progesterone. You may therefore need to avoid gas-producing foods such as cabbage, onions, and corn.

Sugar contains about 45 calories per tablespoon, but has no protein, vitamins, or minerals. These empty calories should have a minimal part in your diet. Sugar can be replaced with fresh fruits and unsweetened juice.

Chemical additives present in processed foods have not all been proven absolutely safe in pregnancy. To be safe, eat as many fresh, unprocessed foods as you can.

**Caffeine Consumption.** Caffeine is a substance found naturally in coffee, tea, cola drinks, and chocolate. It may also be found in certain medications.

Caffeine readily finds its way to the fetus, and the concentration of caffeine in fetal blood will be about the same as the level in the mother's blood. Studies have not shown an association between caffeine consumption and fetal abnormalities, but it is known that caffeine is a powerful stimulant. Caffeine also increases production of stress hormones. This increase causes constriction of uterine blood vessels, which lessens the blood flow to the uterus and temporarily decreases the amount of oxygen reaching the fetus.

Consuming large amounts of caffeine cannot be good for you or your baby. Since this substance has not been proven absolutely safe for the developing baby, it is wise to eliminate, or at least severely restrict, caffeine consumption during pregnancy.

**Artificial Sweeteners.** Little is known about the long-term safety of nonsugar sweeteners, such as saccharin and aspartame. Saccharin has been associated with bladder cancer, and no one is sure about its long-term effects on the developing baby. Aspartame has not been proven unsafe, but there are no long-term studies that show it *is* safe for the developing baby. Perhaps the best advice is to consume these products in moderation or to avoid them altogether during pregnancy.

**Herbal Teas.** Just because herbal teas are considered "natural" does not mean that they are safe for pregnant women. Some herbs and herbal teas contain drugs. Ginseng tea, for example, contains a small amount of estrogen. Teas made from juniper berries may cause stomach irritation. Check with your doctor or pharmacist about the safety of particular herbs and herbal teas before you consume them.

**Weight Control.** Never begin a diet program to lose weight while you are pregnant, unless advised to do so by your doctor. *Never* crash diet. If you reduce your food intake to extremely low levels, you can harm your developing baby. Remember that all of the important nutrients that are critical for your baby's growth must be in your diet.

If you are overweight or gaining weight quite rapidly, your doctor can prescribe a healthy, low-calorie diet that is still in keeping with a healthy pregnancy. He may also have you discuss your diet with a professional dietician so that you may plan specific daily menus.

If you are gaining too little weight during pregnancy, this may also be a cause for concern. A total weight gain of less than 15 pounds during the entire nine months of pregnancy may cause your baby to be abnormally small or growth-retarded. These babies often have a variety of serious problems after birth, such as feeding difficulties and learning disabilities. Furthermore, pregnant women who gain too little weight due to an inadequate diet have a greater chance of developing anemia and preeclampsia.

If you have been **gaining too** little weight, your doctor may perform an ultrasound examination to determine if your lack of weight gain is affecting the growth of the baby. This test will measure the size of the baby's head, chest, and abdomen. By comparing your baby's measurements with those of other normal pregnancies, your doctor can determine if your baby is growing normally.

If you are gaining too little weight, your doctor may advise you to decrease your level of exercise. He will also prescribe a diet that will increase your caloric intake.

One of the best ways to control your weight during pregnancy is to eat according to your appetite. By eating healthy, well-balanced meals, you will help ensure good nutrition for you and your baby. Don't feel that you must eat more than your appetite dictates just because you are pregnant. On the other hand, don't restrict your food intake unless advised to do so by your doctor.

Physical activity is as much a part of weight control as is your caloric intake. Be sure to engage in some form of exercise every day during pregnancy (see *For You and Your Baby*, page 50). It will make you feel better, it will help you control your weight, and it will make getting back into shape after pregnancy easier.

You will find more information on adequate weight gain in the *Ask the Doctor* section on page 24. If you are concerned about your degree of weight gain, talk to your doctor.

**Special Diets.** If you were following any type of special diet—whether to lose weight, to control an illness like diabetes, or to prevent or treat a condition like high blood cholesterol or high blood pressure—be sure to discuss it with your doctor. Now that you are pregnant, you may need to modify it so that you and your baby get enough of the nutrients you both need.

# DAILY FOOD GUIDE

Use the following guide to help you decide if your daily diet is sufficient for pregnancy. Pay specific attention to serving size and to variety in your diet. The sixth column ("Number of Servings You Missed Today") will help you decide if you are getting enough servings of each type of food to meet your daily requirements. Several times during pregnancy, analyze your diet over a period of days.

| FOOD CATEGORY | PRIMARY NUTRIENTS OR NUTRITIVE ROLE | NUMBER OF DAILY SERVINGS | EXAMPLES OF SINGLE SERVINGS |
|---|---|---|---|
| Dairy | Calcium, phosphorus, vitamin D, protein | 4 | 8 oz. milk, 1⅓ cups cottage cheese, 1½ oz. cheese, 1½ cups ice cream |
| High-quality protein | Complete protein, iron, folate, vitamin A, B-complex vitamins | 3 to 4 | 2–3 oz. meat, 2 medium eggs, 8–12 small oysters or clams, 1 cup baked beans or dried peas, ¼ cup peanut butter, ½ cup nuts, 1 cup tofu |
| Grains and breads | B-complex vitamins, incomplete proteins, iron, (also provide energy and fiber) | 4 or more (as needed for calories) | 1 slice bread (whole-grain or enriched), ½ cup cooked cereal, 1 tbsp. wheat germ, ½ cup brown rice or macaroni, 1 tortilla or bagel, 1 pancake (5-inch) |
| Green and yellow vegetables | Vitamin A, folate, vitamin C, vitamin E, riboflavin, iron, magnesium | 1 to 2 | 1 stalk broccoli, 1 small sweet potato, ¾ cup carrots, ½ cup spinach, 3½ oz. romaine, ½ cup squash |
| Citrus fruits; fruits and vegetables rich in vitamin C | Vitamin C, folate | 1 to 2 | 1 orange, ½ cup grapefruit, ½ cup orange juice, ¾ cup strawberries, 1 cup tomato juice, 1 large tomato, ½ green pepper, ¾ cup cabbage |
| Potatoes and other fruits and vegetables | Vitamins (also provide energy and fiber) | 1 or more as needed for calories | 1 potato, ½ cup cauliflower, ½ cup beets, ½ cup corn, ½ cup eggplant, ½ cup celery |
| Fats | Vitamin A, vitamin E (also provide energy) | 1 to 2 | 1 tbsp. oil, fortified margarine, butter, mayonnaise, or salad dressing |
| Fluids | Necessary because of increased metabolic rate (also increases comfort) | 2 to 3 quarts (drink to satisfy thirst) | 1 glass (8 oz.) of water, juice, or other beverage (avoid alcohol and caffeine) |
| Iodine-containing foods | Iodine | Salt to taste at table or in cooking | Iodized salt (avoid excessive amounts), seafood |
| Foods consisting primarily of nonnutritious calories | (Provide energy) | In moderation, and only after daily nutrient requirements have been satisfied | Candy bar, jam, sugar, honey, syrup |

| NUMBER OF SERVINGS YOU HAD TODAY | NUMBER OF SERVINGS YOU MISSED TODAY | FOOD CATEGORY |
|---|---|---|
| | | Dairy |
| | | High-quality protein |
| | | Grains and breads |
| | | Green and yellow vegetables |
| | | Citrus fruits; fruits and vegetables rich in vitamin C |
| | | Potatoes and other fruits and vegetables |
| | | Fats |
| | | Fluids |
| | | Iodine-containing foods |
| | | Foods consisting primarily of nonnutritious calories |

# Your Growing Baby

During the second month after conception, your baby continues to undergo great changes in shape and form. She has the appearance of a living—but not yet clearly human—being. During this month, she will grow about a quarter of an inch each week, and by the end of the month, will weigh one thirtieth of an ounce and be about one-and-one-eighth inches long. Her cells will continue to multiply, grow, fold, and develop into forms that will make up all the parts of her body.

By now, your baby's heart has formed; it is beating a vigorous 60 to 70 times per minute and is forcing fluid through the small blood vessels that are beginning to form.

Even though they won't actually be used for many more months, your baby's lungs are beginning to form in her tiny chest.

Eight to ten vertebrae (bones of the spinal column) have now developed, and your baby's brain, spinal cord, and nerves are well established. The baby's brain is even beginning to send nerve signals to her muscles.

Kidneys that are no larger than the head of a pin are now present and will soon begin the process of making urine. The thyroid and adrenal glands are taking shape and will begin to make hormones that will be necessary for the baby's growth in the months to come. And the stomach, intestines, and liver have taken their proper places in her abdomen.

Baby's external features are starting to take shape, too. Though not looking quite human yet, facial features are now becoming more well defined and ears are beginning to form. Muscles, bones, and skin are also developing rapidly, giving your baby more of a childlike appearance.

Until the end of the second month after conception, your baby is still called an embryo. By the end of the second month, however, all of the organs that she will ever need in her life will have formed, and she will begin a period of rapid growth to eventually become your newborn baby. From this point until delivery, she will be called a fetus.

Throughout the second month, the placenta also undergoes rapid growth and development. Early in the first month, the cells that were destined to form the placenta began to secrete a hormone called human chorionic gonadotropin or HCG. During the first trimester, HCG stimulates your ovaries to produce estrogen and progesterone—the hormones that make it possible for your body to adapt to pregnancy. (Since HCG is produced only when you are pregnant, it is this substance that is detected when a pregnancy test comes back positive.)

Eventually, the placenta itself will be primarily responsible for secreting estrogen and progesterone into your body. Indeed, by the second month, the placenta has already begun churning out increasing amounts of these vital hormones. By the end of the first trimester, the placenta will be developed enough to take over the role of producing all of the estrogen and progesterone needed during pregnancy.

Even though you are not yet aware of it, many amazing things have taken place in your body since conception occurred. A single cell has multiplied into a fetus made up of millions of cells. Your baby is being formed.

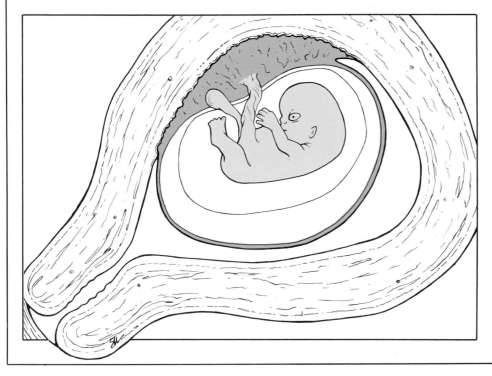

# MONTH

# Your Changing Body

During the second month of pregnancy, you will normally find that you become tired more easily and that you require extra sleep. The daily routines that were so simple before pregnancy now wear you out before the end of the day. This is understandable if you stop to think about all of the changes that are now going on in your body. Your developing baby is taking nutrients and energy from your body, your ovaries are churning out large amounts of hormones, and your body's metabolism is changing rapidly. It takes time for your body to adjust.

If you are a working woman or have young children at home, this may be a very trying time. But you can look forward to the end of your first trimester, when the fatigue and the morning sickness are gone and you discover a renewed sense of energy.

Other discomforts that begin at this time are breast tenderness and a sensation of fullness. They occur because the estrogen and progesterone made by the ovaries and by the developing placenta are preparing the breasts for milk production after you deliver. So whether or not you are planning to nurse your baby, your breasts will enlarge and develop more blood vessels as pregnancy goes on. In most women, breast size increases during pregnancy by at least one whole cup size and by one bra size. For example, bra size may increase from a 34B to a 36C.

These feelings of breast discomfort are similar to those that you may feel immediately before your menstrual period—tingling, throbbing, fullness, and increased sensitivity to touch. Like other common discomforts of early pregnancy, much of your breast tenderness will begin to subside after the end of the third month.

During your second month of pregnancy, there are many changes that are going on in your body, some of which will not be apparent to you. For example, even though you can't see or feel it yet, your uterus is growing rapidly, and by the end of your second month of

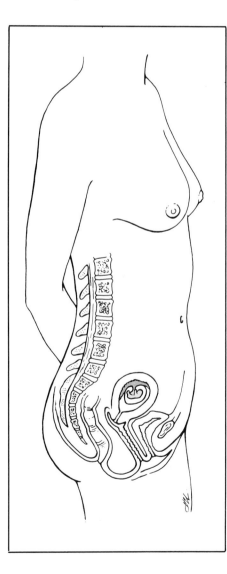

pregnancy, it will be about four times larger than it was before pregnancy. Your cervix (the part of the uterus that protrudes into the vaginal cavity) is enlarging, softening, and turning slightly blue

> Your developing baby takes energy and nutrients from your body, and it takes time for your body to adjust.

in color due to increased growth of blood vessels.

To supply the increasing oxygen and nutrient requirements of the baby and the placenta, the amount of blood being produced in your body increases, and your heart enlarges slightly and beats faster. You will take breaths about two to four times more often per minute and your breathing will be deeper.

Pregnancy changes not only your body but also your emotional state. By the end of the second month, it is common to have self-doubts or even to feel ambivalent toward your baby. You may be unhappy that you are pregnant or you may begin to doubt your ability to care for your newborn child. At one moment you may cry or be angry and in another feel joy and dedication. If you are acting differently than you usually do, be assured that these changes are not abnormal.

# How Much Weight Should I Gain?

A certain amount of weight gain—coupled with proper nutrition—is now expected and required to ensure both your health and the health of your baby.

From the early 1950s until the early 1970s, pregnant women were advised to gain only ten to 15 pounds during pregnancy. It was thought that by limiting weight gain in the mother, the baby's weight could be kept low. This, in turn, was supposed to reduce the problems associated with delivering a large baby and cut down on the amount of weight the mother would have to lose after delivery.

Today, however, recommendations for proper weight gain during pregnancy have changed—mainly because of concern over the effects of poor weight gain on the developing baby. A certain amount of weight gain—coupled with proper nutrition—is now expected and required to ensure both your health and the health of your baby. Your doctor, therefore, will check your weight during each office visit to make certain that you are not gaining too much or too little.

**Optimal Weight Gain.** The optimal weight gain during pregnancy for an average-sized woman carrying a single baby is 24 to 30 pounds. If you were underweight before you became pregnant, you will probably be encouraged to gain closer to 30 pounds, and if you were previously over-

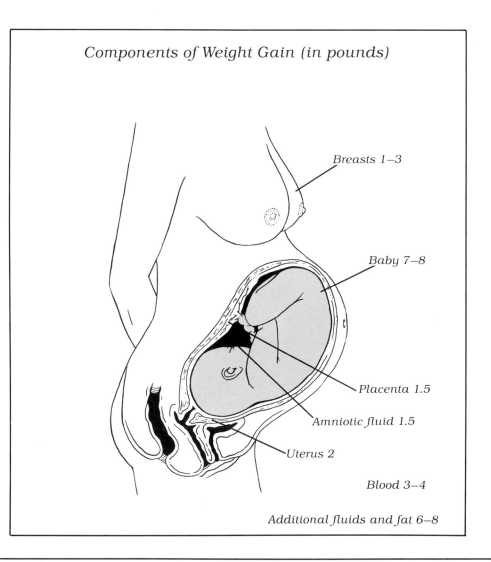

*Components of Weight Gain (in pounds)*

Breasts 1–3

Baby 7–8

Placenta 1.5

Amniotic fluid 1.5

Uterus 2

Blood 3–4

Additional fluids and fat 6–8

weight, you will probably be advised to gain closer to 20 pounds.

During the first trimester, your weight gain will probably be between zero and four pounds. Because of morning sickness, some women gain no weight and may even lose one to two pounds. This slight weight loss is not abnormal and will not harm the baby at this stage.

During the second trimester, you will normally gain from 11 to 14 pounds, and during the third trimester, an additional 11 to 13 pounds. Another way to look at this is that after the first trimester, you will gain about one pound each week.

The best time to weigh yourself is first thing in the morning when you rise from bed (if you have to urinate, do so before you weigh yourself). Many women will find that they weigh one to three pounds more at night than they did in the morning. This additional weight gain during the day is caused by retention of water, usually in the legs. When you lie down at night, this excess water will reenter your bloodstream and be eliminated in your urine the next morning. For this reason, what you weigh in the morning is considered to be your true weight.

It is extremely important to note that while gaining enough weight is essential, you need to be sure that you are providing you and your baby with the nutrients you both need. To learn more about proper nutrition, see the section entitled *For You and Your Baby* on page 16.

**Where Does the Weight Go?**
Some of the weight gained in pregnancy is accounted for by the growth of your baby and some is accounted for by the changes in your body that are necessary to support the pregnancy. During the last month of pregnancy with an average-sized baby, your weight is distributed in the following way:

- Baby . . . . . . . . . . 7-8 pounds
- Placenta . . . . . . . 1½ pounds
- Amniotic fluid . . . 1½ pounds
- Increase in weight of uterus . . . . . . . . 2 pounds
- Increase in weight of mother's blood . 3-4 pounds
- Increase in weight of breasts . . . . . 1-3 pounds

The remaining six to eight pounds is accounted for by the increased fat tissue and fluid that have accumulated in the mother. Most of the fat is carried in the hips and thighs.

**Too Much Weight Gain.** Weight gain in excess of 40 pounds will, in itself, have little significant effect on your pregnancy. Your baby will not grow much larger than he would had you gained a more moderate 25 pounds. Indeed, women who gain even 80 to 100 pounds during their pregnancies frequently have babies that weigh seven to eight pounds.

The major problem with excessive weight gain during pregnancy is what it does to your body. Backaches, leg pain, cramps, and stretch marks occur sooner and may be more severe if you gain excessive weight. On the other hand, with a more moderate weight gain, you're likely to look better, feel better, and have fewer aches and pains. Additionally, the more excessive your weight gain during pregnancy, the harder it will be to take the weight off after delivery.

Sudden, excessive weight gain—that is, a weight gain of two to ten pounds over a period of one to three days—is a warning sign that may indicate preeclampsia (toxemia), a serious condition associated with high blood pressure and seizures. If you experience a rapid weight gain over a period of only a few days, call your doctor immediately.

**Too Little Weight Gain.** A total weight gain of less than 15 pounds during pregnancy may cause low birth weight and growth retardation in your baby. Such babies may develop mental retardation or learning disabilities later in life.

## This Month's Visit

During this month's office visit, the doctor will probably:

- Check your weight. By now, you may have gained about one to two pounds.
- Check your blood pressure. Your blood pressure should be the same as it was before pregnancy.
- Check your urine for sugar and protein. You should normally have no sugar or protein in your urine.
- Ask about symptoms of pregnancy. By now, you will probably be experiencing morning sickness, frequent urination, and breast tenderness.
- Ask how you are feeling. Tell your doctor about any unusual symptoms that you have noticed.
- Check the growth of the uterus by doing a pelvic examination. By now, the uterus will be about four times larger than it was before pregnancy.
- Examine the fallopian tubes and ovaries. They should not grow in size during a normal pregnancy.
- Explain to you the results of the laboratory tests performed at your last visit. Your doctor will be able to tell you your blood type, blood count, immunity to German measles, and the results of the Pap smear. No new tests need to be performed this month, unless you are ill or have developed complications.
- If necessary, give you prescriptions for the relief of pregnancy symptoms. During early pregnancy, it is best to take no medication other than iron and vitamins. But if you have severe nausea and vomiting, for example, your doctor may prescribe certain safe medications to make you more comfortable.

# Getting off to a Good Start

These suggestions, coupled with your doctor's instructions, can help you deal with the physical and emotional discomforts that commonly occur in the first trimester.

Pregnancy should be a happy and healthy time in your life. It is a natural process that can bring you a deep sense of contentment and joy. But because pregnancy involves so many physical and emotional changes, it can also bring with it some common discomforts and concerns.

Only a few decades ago, these discomforts were considered to be unavoidable consequences of childbearing. Today, however, we know that many of them can be minimized and sometimes treated with good prenatal care, allowing you to get that much more pleasure out of your pregnancy.

Since pregnancy is customarily divided into three segments or trimesters, the discomforts you may experience will be discussed in relation to the trimester in which they are most likely to occur. In this *Coping with the Changes* section, therefore, you will find suggestions for dealing with the physical discomforts, emotions, and concerns that you're likely to experience during the first three months of your pregnancy (you'll find similar *Coping* sections for the second and third trimesters). These suggestions, coupled with

your doctor's instructions and advice, can help you start your pregnancy off right.

## COMMON DISCOMFORTS OF THE FIRST TRIMESTER

During the first six weeks or so of pregnancy, the physical changes you experience are due primarily to your increasing hormone levels. Sometimes these early changes are subtle; so subtle, in fact, that if it weren't for your missed menstrual period, you might not even realize that you are pregnant.

After the first six weeks, however, some of the physical changes you experience will be caused by the growth of the baby. These changes will become more noticeable as the baby gets larger and larger. Although the most obvious changes occur in your uterus and abdomen, pregnancy affects almost every organ of your body. Keeping these changes in mind, it is easier to understand why certain discomforts occur.

The following practical suggestions may help you ease the common discomforts of the first trimester. You need to remember, however, that you should avoid

taking any medication or home remedy unless it is specifically recommended by your doctor. If you have any questions, be sure to consult him.

**Fatigue.** Fatigue and the need for extra sleep occur in nearly every pregnancy, mostly during the first trimester. Listen to your body and treat fatigue with rest as often as you can. If you work, schedule rest periods at regular intervals throughout the day. Don't ever try to fight your fatigue with stimulants such as coffee or "pep pills."

**Breast Tenderness.** As the breasts enlarge under the influence of your increasing hormone levels, they will become sensitive and tender. Starting in the early months of pregnancy, begin wearing a well-fitting, supportive bra during the day. You may even wish to wear the bra while sleeping if it seems to help. Cold towels applied for a few minutes several times a day may also help to ease discomfort. Pads worn underneath the bra will help prevent colostrum from staining your clothing.

**Frequent Urination.** As the enlarging uterus presses up against the bladder and decreases the bladder's capacity, you will have

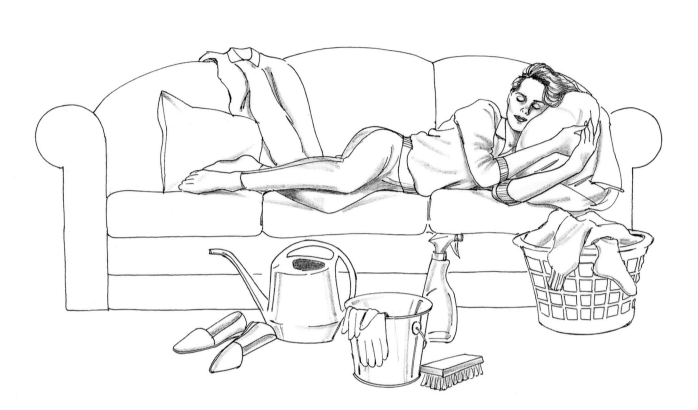

the urge to urinate more frequently. This is a normal and unavoidable symptom of early pregnancy. There are, however, ways to decrease the inconvenience of frequent urination.

If your sleep is disturbed by your frequent need to urinate, you might try not drinking any liquids within the two to three hours before bedtime. Also, be sure to empty your bladder completely before traveling in a car, train, or bus, where facilities may not be available or may be inconvenient to use.

If your urination is extremely frequent (more than once an hour) or if pain or burning occurs, call your doctor, since these may be signs of a bladder infection.

**Morning Sickness.** About two-thirds of all pregnant women experience nausea and vomiting during the first trimester. These symptoms usually disappear without treatment by about the fourth month of pregnancy.

Nausea and vomiting are often triggered by an empty stomach, certain foods and food odors, and fatigue. Here are a few suggestions you might try in order to increase your comfort until morning sickness passes.

- Put some dry crackers by your bed at night and eat them in the morning before you get out of bed.
- Eat high-protein foods throughout the day. This prevents a drop in your blood sugar level, which is thought to be linked to nausea.
- Eat five light meals a day instead of three large meals so that your stomach is never empty.
- Carry a high-carbohydrate snack (such as fresh fruit, bread, or crackers) with you during the day and eat it when you begin to feel nauseated.
- Eliminate fatty food, spicy food, fried food, and caffeine from your diet during the first trimester. All of these tend to irritate the stomach.
- Avoid odors that you know will make you nauseated. For example, if the smell of frying food makes you queasy, you can eliminate some of these cooking odors by eating more cold foods.
- Drink fluids between meals instead of with meals. Sometimes, separating food and liquids improves digestion.

• Take your prenatal vitamins, which are often irritating to the stomach, with your largest meal.

If these measures do not ease your nausea and vomiting, let your doctor know, since he can prescribe a safe medication to relieve your symptoms. Remember, however, that it's safest to try to control these problems through dietary changes; medications should be used as a last resort.

Severe, frequent, or protracted vomiting should be reported to your doctor immediately, since this may be a sign of a more serious problem, such as appendicitis.

**Constipation.** This is a common complaint during pregnancy. It is usually the result of the relaxation of the smooth muscle in your digestive tract and the pressure of the enlarging uterus on the rectum. Constipation may be aggravated by iron supplements, lack of adequate fluid intake, and inactivity. The following tips may help you relieve constipation.

• Increase the fiber in your diet by eating more leafy vegetables and whole grain cereals and breads.
• Drink two to three quarts of liquid each day. This will help to keep your stool soft.
• Exercise—even if it's only walking—every day.
• Include fruits that have a laxative effect, like prunes, raisins, and figs, in your diet.
• Try having a bowel movement at the same time each day.

If these measures are unsuccessful, ask your doctor to suggest a mild laxative or stool softener that you can purchase at the drugstore without a prescription. Never take mineral oil, since this can block the absorption of certain vitamins in your stomach. Never use an enema unless approved by your doctor.

**Vaginal Discharge.** A thin, milky-white to yellowish vaginal discharge is common throughout pregnancy. Like most other discom-

forts during the early months of pregnancy, this is caused by your increasing levels of hormones. If this discharge bothers you, cleanse the skin outside your vagina with a mild soap-and-water solution two

---

## Maintaining a positive attitude may help you to relieve some of the physical discomforts of pregnancy.

---

or three times a day. Never douche unless directed to do so by your doctor. Wear cotton undergarments, which will help to keep the skin outside the vagina dry and prevent irritation. You may also want to wear a panty liner to prevent the discharge from staining your clothing.

If your vaginal discharge is heavy or if it causes itching or burning, notify your doctor, since these may be signs of a vaginal infection.

### PSYCHOLOGICAL CHANGES

Pregnancy is a time of growth, change, enrichment, and challenge. It is a time when you will confront your fears and expectations about becoming a parent. It is a rare woman who does not notice significant emotional changes throughout her pregnancy.

Although there are certain similarities in all pregnancies, each pregnancy is special. Shifts in your body image, changes in your hormones, and your attitude toward cultural pressures and expectations will all combine to make your experience of pregnancy unique.

Each of the physical landmarks of pregnancy is accompanied by specific psychological issues that will affect your perception of that particular part of your pregnancy. For example, if your pregnancy was planned and wished for, you and your partner will probably respond with joy and anticipation to the news that you have conceived. If, on the other hand, the pregnancy was unexpected, you may initially have mixed feelings or may even be angry.

Interactions between your mind and your body will occur throughout your pregnancy. For example, a high level of stress in your life or negative feelings about being pregnant may contribute to some of the nausea that occurs in the first trimester. Conversely, the nausea and vomiting may make you feel less than enthusiastic about being pregnant. The important thing to remember is that since your body and mind interact in this way during pregnancy, trying to maintain a positive attitude may help to alleviate some physical discomforts.

Numerous psychological changes will occur the moment that you become aware that you are pregnant. Although you may not look any different to other people for weeks to come, chances are you'll start to feel different from the very beginning. Your usual emotional highs and lows will be magnified at this time, and if this is your first pregnancy, these feelings may confuse you. Things that normally would not bother you may provoke you to tears or cause you to become depressed or angry, even at people you care about.

These sudden emotional swings are more pronounced in some women than in others. Your reactions will depend, in part, on your personality structure, the kind of stress that you are experiencing, and the emotional support that you are receiving, as well as on the hormonal changes occurring in your body.

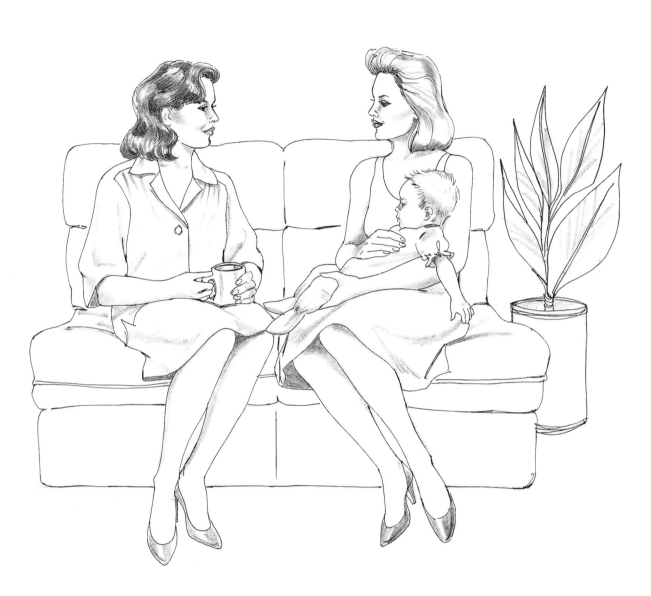

Since the risk of miscarriage approaches 20 percent in the first trimester, you may worry about whether the pregnancy will continue. If you had a previous miscarriage, this will be a time of heightened stress and anxiety.

Talking to a counselor or to a friend who has been pregnant might be very helpful at this time, especially if the feelings of anxiety and tension appear to be signifi-

cantly interfering with your daily activities. Also, it is important to try to get as much rest as you can during the first trimester because rest will make you feel better.

If there is a lot of stress in your life, you may want to try to modify or avoid as much of it as you can (for example, you may want to have relatives or friends—as well as your husband—help with chores and errands if you have too little energy

and too many demands on your time). You may also want to learn some relaxation techniques to help you cope with the stress that you feel.

Be assured that certain emotional changes in pregnancy are normal and will eventually pass as pregnancy progresses.

Your partner may also undergo significant emotional changes during your pregnancy. Although there is no physical basis for this, it is nevertheless very real and, to some degree, predictable. Men, as well as women, bring to a pregnancy their own perceptions about the mechanics and significance of pregnancy, birth, and parenthood. How the father-to-be perceived his own parents can directly affect his feelings about becoming a parent himself. For some men, being able to father a child may create a sense of heightened self-esteem or masculinity. On the other hand, if there was a history of poor family relations or a missing father, some men may view pregnancy with ambivalence or even fear.

For the future father, there is no internal reality—no physical transformation to feel. The only way that he can experience your pregnancy is through what you tell him. Perhaps not until he can place his hand on your stomach and feel the baby's movements will the father perceive the fetus as a growing child.

Participating in prenatal doctor visits may be one way to allow the father to have a greater awareness of the reality of pregnancy. If an ultrasound study is performed, viewing the ultrasound pictures can be an invaluable experience because on the screen the father will have a visual confirmation of the existence of your pregnancy.

It is still difficult for some men to admit openly that they have concerns, fears, and perhaps even ambivalent feelings about their partner's pregnancy; yet these feelings are nearly universal. Many men even develop certain physical symptoms in relation to a pregnancy, such as nausea, headache, and backache. These symptoms tend to appear by the beginning of the second trimester. There may also be increased feelings of anxiety and depression.

The father-to-be's tasks during the first trimester should include both learning to accept the pregnancy and providing emotional

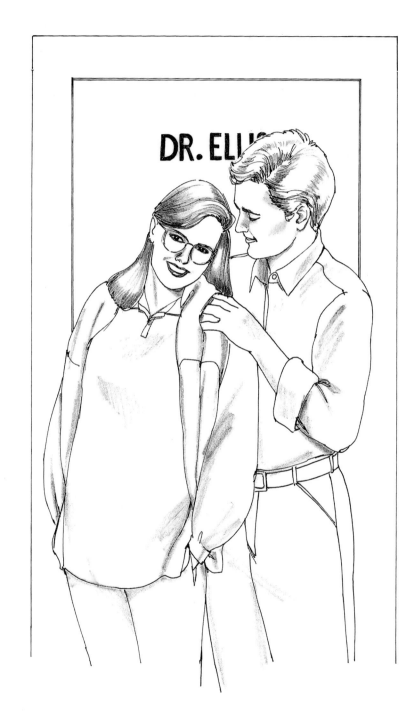

support to his partner. Many men are ecstatic about the prospect of becoming a father, but some may be frightened by this as well. The mother-to-be plays a role in shaping her partner's attitude and initial reaction, but mutual support, open lines of communication, and reassurance are the responsibilities of both parents.

As a couple, you are now sharing fears, needs, and joys that you may have never experienced before. But because you are unique, your emotional responses will be unique. It is important to support each other throughout pregnancy with acceptance and love.

## SEXUAL RELATIONS

Your feelings about your own sexuality and your desire for sexual activity may also change during this time. Sometimes, pregnancy alters a couple's sexual desires, which can lead to feelings of frustration and anxiety unless both partners understand the reasons for the change. Keep in mind that your emotions and desires, your comfort, and the safety of both mother and baby—rather than some abstract norm—should guide your sexual activites during pregnancy.

The different stages of pregnancy can affect a woman in different ways. Many women report a diminished desire for sex in the first trimester because of fatigue, nausea, and sore breasts. On the other hand, some women actually feel a surge of interest in sexual relations. For these women, any fears and doubts about their ability to conceive have been relieved and they now feel more comfortable and relaxed.

A virtually universal fear is concern about injuring the developing baby during intercourse. In most instances, intercourse is safe up until the time when the amniotic sac breaks. If you have a history of previous miscarriages or other complications or if you are experiencing complications with your current pregnancy, your doctor may advise that you restrict intercourse during part or all of your pregnancy. If you have any concerns about the safety of sexual intercourse during pregnancy, be sure to discuss them with your doctor.

## SAFEGUARDING YOUR BABY'S HEALTH

The first trimester is a time when the developing baby's organs and tissues are beginning to form. This is also a time in which she is most vulnerable to certain substances and environmental hazards.

The environment in which your baby undergoes her rapid development is extremely important. For many years it was thought that the placenta kept all dangerous agents from passing into the baby's bloodstream, thus protecting her from harmful substances to which the mother was exposed. Unfortunately, this is now known to be untrue. Virtually anything that is eaten, inhaled, injected, or contracted by the mother will eventually enter the baby's body via the placenta. For this reason, you must be extremely cautious about exposure to any substances that may be hazardous to your baby.

**Infectious Diseases.** During the first trimester you must be extremely careful to avoid being exposed to certain infectious diseases. Although most common infectious diseases, such as colds and the flu, will have no effect on pregnancy, some diseases that may be caught from others can have very serious effects on the developing baby.

The herpes virus is responsible for frequent, painful ulcers that may occur in the genital areas of both men and women. This virus is sexually transmitted; it is spread by direct contact with the genital organs. This infection rarely causes serious problems in the woman; however, the newborn baby may become infected and die if she comes into contact with an open herpes ulcer in the mother's genital region during delivery. For this reason, cesarean section is performed if a woman has a herpes ulcer in the genital region when she goes into labor. If you or your partner have had herpes, it is important that you tell your doctor; he will then carefully examine your genital area during prenatal visits.

> You must be extremely careful to avoid exposure to any potentially harmful substance during pregnancy.

Syphilis is another sexually transmitted disease that may seriously affect the baby. If the mother develops an active syphilis infection during pregnancy, the bacteria may enter the baby's bloodstream and cause a variety of abnormalities, including malformations of the heart, eyes, bones, and mouth. Therefore, a blood test to detect the presence of syphilis is usually part of the routine blood testing performed on a pregnant woman at her first prenatal visit. If a pregnant woman thinks that she may have caught syphilis during pregnancy, she should tell her doctor immediately.

Rubella (German measles) is a common infectious disease that usually affects children. The rash and fever of rubella usually pass within a few days, and complete recovery from the infection is the rule. Rubella infection during pregnancy, however, may have serious effects on the baby, especially if the infection develops early in pregnancy when the organs of the fetus are just beginning to form. Complications in the baby may include microcephaly (abnormally small head), mental retardation, seizures, eye defects, heart malformations, and deafness.

If a pregnant woman suspects that she may have come into contact with someone with rubella, she should report it to her doctor immediately, even if a rash or fever has not yet appeared. The doctor may then perform blood tests to determine if the woman has actually caught rubella.

A woman who is considering becoming pregnant should be tested to see if she is immune to rubella. Usually, if a person has had rubella at one time in her life, she will never get the infection again. If a woman is not immune, most doctors advise that she obtain a rubella vaccination before becoming pregnant.

Toxoplasmosis is another infection that may have serious effects on the baby. The mother may become infected with the toxoplasmosis organism if she eats raw infected meat or if she is in close contact with infected cats.

Babies born to infected mothers may have many serious birth defects, including microcephaly, seizures, and disorders of the brain, liver, blood, lungs, and kidneys.

To avoid infection with toxoplasmosis, you should always cook meat thoroughly, never eat rare meat, and avoid contact with cat litter boxes during pregnancy.

**Radiation.** All forms of radiation are potentially hazardous to your developing baby, especially during the first trimester. For this reason, you should avoid any exposure to radiation if you know or suspect that you are pregnant.

The effect of radiation on the developing baby depends on the amount of radiation, the length of exposure, and how far along you are in your pregnancy. If you need to have X rays performed—to detect an injury such as a broken bone,

for example—make certain that you inform the X-ray technician that you are pregnant. A lead shield will then be placed over your abdomen to protect the baby. Since X rays cannot penetrate lead, your baby will be safe.

If X rays or any form of radiation are used where you work, you will need to ask for reassignment to another area or take a leave of absence for the duration of your pregnancy.

X rays used in airport security systems will not harm your baby since the level of radiation they produce is very low and the exposure time is short.

**Cigarettes.** Cigarette smoking poses a serious threat to the well-being of your baby. Mothers who smoke have smaller babies than mothers who do not smoke; these low-birth-weight babies are more likely to suffer from a variety of problems after birth. Smoking is

also associated with a greater incidence of miscarriage, prematurity, stillbirth, and death of the baby soon after birth. If you smoke, stop immediately—for your baby's sake as well as for yours.

**Marijuana.** The use of marijuana during pregnancy may also pose a threat to the developing baby. Marijuana use has been associated with prolonged labor, precipitate delivery (rapid expulsion of the baby), low birth weight, prematurity, and a greater risk that the baby will not get enough oxygen via the placenta.

**Cocaine.** Cocaine has profound effects on the pregnant woman and her baby. It causes an increase in the mother's heart rate; constriction of blood vessels in the placenta, which allows less blood to reach the baby; increased secretion of stress hormones in the mother, which causes constriction of blood vessels in the uterus; and abnor-

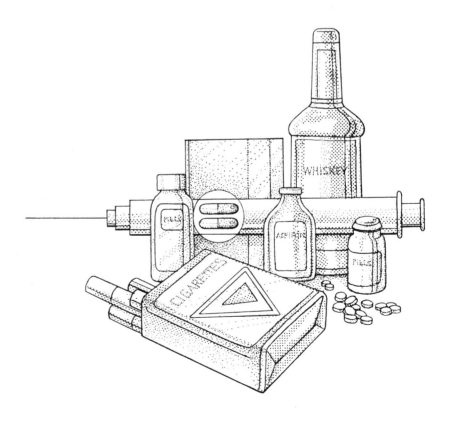

mally strong uterine contractions. Cocaine use is also thought to be related to a higher incidence of miscarriage and to separation of the placenta from the wall of the uterus before delivery. Infants whose mothers used cocaine often have a difficult time adjusting to environmental stimuli after birth and may be addicted to the drug.

**Alcohol.** Even moderate (one or two drinks per day) and social (three to four drinks per day) drinking have been associated with fetal alcohol syndrome. Affected babies are born with physical malformations, including microcephaly, certain heart defects, and mental retardation. No safe level of alcohol consumption has been established for pregnancy. As a result, it is best to avoid alcohol consumption during pregnancy. If you have any questions about alcohol consumption, discuss them with your doctor.

**Other Medications and Drugs.** Since most drugs have not been proven absolutely safe for use during pregnancy and since some drugs are known to be hazardous, you will need to be extremely cautious about using any medication during pregnancy.

Drugs that can alter the baby's development and cause abnormalities are called teratogens. Teratogens are especially dangerous to the developing baby during the first trimester, when the major organ systems are forming.

Many specific drugs have been identified as being hazardous to the developing baby. In some cases, their effects are severe; for example, they may prevent the formation of the baby's arms and legs or they may cause heart defects or a cleft lip. In other cases, the effect may be relatively mild and treatable; for example, a drug taken by the mother may cause anemia (an abnormally low level of oxygen-carrying blood cells) in the newborn.

Since most drugs have not been proven safe for use during

pregnancy, it is always best to avoid taking any medication unless it is absolutely necessary for your health or the health of the baby. During pregnancy, drugs should be used only to treat a serious illness that threatens you or your baby or to treat discomforts of pregnancy when all other methods fail. Since the vast majority of discomforts that you will experience in pregnancy are harmless and can often be minimized through nondrug means, you need to weigh the potential risks and benefits of drug use carefully. Never take any prescription drug during pregnancy without first consulting your doctor.

Even certain common medications that are sold without a prescription in drugstores may have a harmful effect on the

developing baby. For example, aspirin may cause problems with blood clotting in the newborn if it is taken by the mother within several days of labor (see *Coping*, page 65, for more on aspirin and other pain relievers). Nasal sprays used to treat sinus congestion may raise a woman's blood pressure and may cause abnormalities in the flow of blood to the placenta. For these reasons, never use a nonprescription drug for any reason without first consulting your doctor.

During your first prenatal visit, your doctor will ask you about medications that you may currently be taking. If you are not sure what they are, bring along the prescription bottles. Your doctor can then determine if the drug will have any dangerous effect on the baby.

## Tips for Kicking the Smoking Habit

When you're pregnant, you want to do everything you can to ensure that your baby is born healthy. If you're a smoker, the best thing that you can do is to stop smoking—now.

You may never have more reasons to quit smoking than you do now that you're pregnant. You can use your baby's health, as well as your own, as your motivation. In addition, there are a variety of tips and techniques that you can use to help you kick the habit.

Begin by recording the number of cigarettes you smoke each day, when you smoke them, and what you're doing when you have each one. Then review the record and try to pinpoint why you smoke each cigarette and what types of activities you associate with smoking. For example, you may find that you tend to smoke after meals or during coffee breaks. You may also find that you tend to light up when you are bored, fidgety, or tense.

The next step is to rearrange your schedule or substitute other

activities for smoking. The following suggestions may help.

- If you smoke during coffee breaks, try substituting a brisk walk or other form of physical activity. This may help you to fight the urge to light up, and it can help you increase your fitness. If it's the coffee itself that you associate with smoking, try switching to a beverage that's healthier for you and your baby, such as juice or water.

- If you tend to smoke after meals, avoid lingering at the table after you finish eating. Try going for a stroll, clearing the table, or making a list of things you'll need when your baby arrives.

- If you smoke when you're bored or fidgety, try taking up a hobby, like knitting or drawing, to keep busy. If you miss handling a cigarette, try playing with coins or marbles, or munch on celery or carrots.

- If you smoke to relieve tension, try taking a walk, practicing your breathing exercises, or picturing how cute and cuddly your healthy baby will be.

# Your Growing Baby

Your baby's third month brings new growth, further development of organs, and more physical activity. By the end of the month, your baby will have grown to about three inches in length and will weigh about one ounce.

During this month, your baby's head will be enlarging rapidly. Her face will become even more human in appearance as her ears and mouth continue to form. Her eyelids, which are just now developing, are tightly closed and will remain sealed for at least three more months. Even now, all the structures needed for your baby's eyesight—the cornea, lens, and retina—are being molded from specialized cells. Parts of her mouth and throat are also coming together; this will enable her to suck and swallow in the coming months. Tiny buds that will develop into baby teeth are just being formed, and distinct lips are appearing.

Your baby's tiny hands are now fully formed, as are her fingers and

---

## Your baby can now kick her legs, make a fist, and open her mouth.

---

fingernails. As her cells continue to multiply and grow, your baby's bones and muscles strengthen. She can now move around easily in her amniotic sac, exercising her new muscles and using her newly formed nervous system to direct her muscles to make these movements. Your baby can now kick her legs, make a fist, turn her head, open her mouth, and squint her face—but she is still too small for you to feel.

The sex of your baby is not yet apparent on the outside, even though it was already determined during the fertilization of your egg. Only by looking at certain sex organs within the baby's body would you be able to tell the sex of your baby at this time.

Your baby's internal organs are continuing to rapidly grow and mature. By the end of her third month, all of her organs will be formed and ready or nearly ready to function. The heart has grown rapidly and is now beating and pumping blood through a simple system of blood vessels. Within weeks, all of the major blood vessels in her body will have reached their final form. Blood now being produced in your baby's bone marrow will be needed in the weeks ahead to supply oxygen to all parts of her rapidly growing body.

Other organs in your baby's body are also beginning to function. Her kidneys are starting to produce small amounts of urine, her brain is sending nerve impulses throughout her body, and her glands are beginning to produce hormones.

Over a three-month period, your baby has grown from a single cell into a clearly human being with organs that now perform complex functions. Your baby's perfect development up to this point has involved a delicate series of steps. Since her tissues and organs are growing at a tremendous rate, she needs constant support from your body—in the forms of proper nutrition and avoidance of harmful substances such as nicotine, alcohol, and other drugs—to provide the building blocks for her continued normal development.

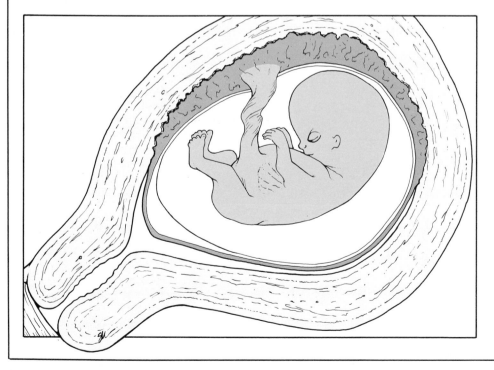

# MONTH

# Your Changing Body

In your third month of pregnancy, your body continues to undergo dramatic changes in response to your increasing levels of hormones and your rapidly enlarging uterus. Certain new discomforts begin at this time and tend to remain until the end of your pregnancy.

By now, you have probably started having problems with constipation. There are several normal changes that your body goes through in pregnancy that may lead to constipation. First, pressure from your enlarging uterus will cause crowding of the digestive organs. This pressure may make it more difficult for stool to pass. Second, increasing levels of the hormone progesterone cause the muscles in the walls of your intestines to contract less strongly, thus slowing the passage of stool from your body. Finally, constipation is a common side effect of the iron tablets that your doctor probably prescribed to supplement your diet. Constipation is generally a problem throughout pregnancy, but fortunately it can be easily treated (see *Coping*, p. 28).

Also beginning in the third month of pregnancy, most women will notice an increased amount of vaginal discharge. This discharge is usually thin, milky white to yellowish in color, odorless, and nonirritating. This discharge is caused by your increasing levels of estrogen and progesterone, which stimulate the cells of the cervix and vagina to produce increased amounts of mucus. Though most of this mucus escapes from the vagina, some remains within the canal of the cervix and hardens to produce the so-called "mucous plug." This hardened mucus seals off the entrance of the cervix for the remainder of pregnancy and is thought to possibly prevent bacteria and other organisms from entering the uterus. Several hours to days before you go into labor, this mucous plug will come loose from the cervix and may be expelled from your vagina.

Since you are more likely to develop certain common vaginal

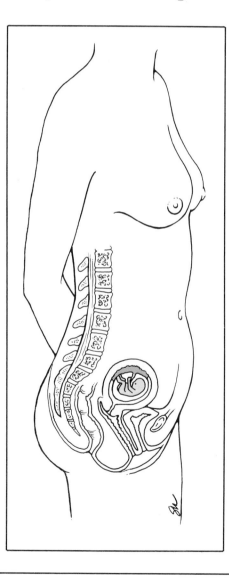

infections during pregnancy, it is important for you to be able to tell the difference between the normal discharge of pregnancy and the

---

### Constipation is a common discomfort throughout pregnancy.

---

discharge caused by infection. In general, the discharge caused by an infection is heavier, dark yellow to green in color, itchy or irritating, and often marked by an unpleasant odor. If you suspect that you have a vaginal infection, you should check with your doctor right away.

Your breasts will also undergo further changes at this time, again in response to the increasing levels of estrogen and progesterone being produced by the placenta. The areolae—the dark skin around your nipples—will enlarge and darken. In preparation for milk production, your breasts will begin to produce a milky white substance called colostrum. During your third month of pregnancy, small amounts of colostrum can actually be expressed from the breasts by gently squeezing the nipple.

Toward the end of the first trimester, it is also common for pregnant women to become more introspective. You may ask yourself "Is this really the best time to be pregnant?" or "Will my baby love me?" Keep in mind that it takes time to accept your new and special role as a mother, and your introspection during pregnancy is a step toward that acceptance.

# Will Heartburn Make My Baby's Hair Grow?

There are a great many "wive's tales" that you may hear when you're pregnant— and most of them aren't true.

Now that you are pregnant, well-meaning individuals are probably giving you advice about things you must do and things you must avoid. There are a great number of "wive's tales" that you may hear during your pregnancy. Although many of these tales have been passed down from generation to generation, most of them are simply not true.

The following are some of the common myths of pregnancy—and the medical reasons why you shouldn't believe them. If you've been given advice about diet, activity, or any other aspect of pregnancy from a relative, friend, or acquaintance, or if you've read or heard a pregnancy "tip" that you're not sure is correct, be certain to discuss it with your doctor.

*If you have heartburn, your baby will have a lot of hair when she is born.*

NOT TRUE: Heartburn during pregnancy is usually caused by the uterus pushing up on your stomach. Nothing you do can affect the growth of your baby's hair. Some babies are born with a full head of hair while others are born nearly bald.

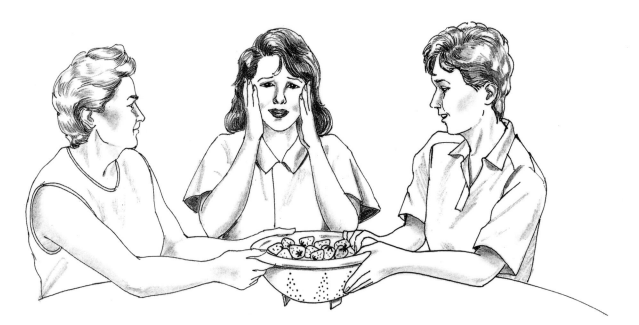

*If you eat strawberries, your baby will develop a strawberry birthmark on her face.*

NOT TRUE: These birthmarks may develop in some babies, but the reason is not known.

*During pregnancy, you must eat a great deal more food because you're "eating for two."*

NOT TRUE: Eat according to your appetite. Remember that the "other person" you're eating for is a tiny being. Gaining too much weight will increase your aches and pains and will make getting back in shape after delivery more difficult. Concentrate, instead, on providing both you and your baby with the nutrients you both need for a healthy pregnancy. Your doctor will watch your weight and advise you if you are gaining too much or too little.

*Do not eat salt because you will develop toxemia (preeclampsia).*

NOT TRUE: Your intake of salt does not cause toxemia (a serious condition marked by very high blood pressure). The cause of toxemia is not known.

*If you wash your hair, your baby will develop pneumonia.*

NOT TRUE: You may continue to wash your hair, shower, and bathe as usual. Even if you do develop a "cold," this cannot be transmitted to your baby.

*If you take a bath or swim, your baby will drown.*

NOT TRUE: The baby is already floating around in the amniotic fluid; she will not drown. Furthermore, water does not enter the vagina, even when you bathe or swim.

*Lifting your arms above your head will cause your baby to be strangled by the umbilical cord.*

NOT TRUE: Some babies do wrap themselves in the umbilical cord as they twist and turn in the uterus, but this has nothing to do

with your arms. Stretching your arms above your head is actually a good exercise during pregnancy.

*If you become mean or angry, your baby will have a bad disposition.*

NOT TRUE: Your emotions will not affect your baby while she is still in your uterus.

*If you play classical music during your pregnancy, your baby will grow up to be an artist.*

NOT TRUE: Your baby may become an artist, but not because you played certain types of music during pregnancy. Soft music will, however, be soothing to the baby; you may even notice that her kicking slows down in response to the music.

*You can predict the baby's sex by the way you carry the baby and by the rate of the baby's heartbeat.*

NOT TRUE: The way you will carry your baby—far in front or close to your body—is related to your baby's position and size and the strength of your abdominal muscles—not to his or her sex. The baby's heart rate may vary from day to day, but on average, the heart rate is the same for boys and girls.

*It is best for you and your baby if you gain very little weight during pregnancy.*

NOT TRUE: Too little weight gain may retard your baby's growth and may cause other serious problems after birth. You should normally gain about 24 to 30 pounds during pregnancy (see page 24).

*Mopping the floor or eating spicy food will make you go into labor.*

NOT TRUE: If you go into labor after doing either of these two, it is purely coincidence. There is nothing that you can do to start your labor.

Once again, if you ever have questions about what you have heard, ask your doctor.

---

## This Month's Visit

During this month's office visit, your doctor will probably:

- Check your weight. By now, you will have gained about two to four pounds.
- Check your blood pressure. This should be the same as it was before pregnancy.
- Check your urine for sugar and protein. There should normally be neither in your urine.
- Ask about symptoms of pregnancy. By now, most of the discomforts of early pregnancy will be subsiding; however, you may now have constipation and an increased vaginal discharge.
- Ask about how you are feeling. Inform your doctor of any physical or emotional feelings that you are having.
- Check the growth of the uterus by either a pelvic examination or by feeling your lower abdomen. By the end of the third month, the top of your uterus will be slightly above the pubic bone.
- Check for your baby's heartbeat. Close to the end of the third month, you and your doctor will be able to hear the heartbeat with an instrument called a doppler. This device uses sound waves to detect faint sounds such as the baby's heartbeat.
- Give you practical advice about the second trimester of pregnancy. Your doctor will probably discuss proper exercise and tell you what types of activities to avoid. This is a good time to ask about how long you can expect to work and how long you can travel.
- Prescribe medications for discomforts such as constipation.
- Perform no new tests.

# Work and Travel During Pregnancy

In general, a pregnant woman is allowed to continue working and traveling throughout pregnancy unless doing so would be hazardous to her or her baby.

## WORKING THROUGH PREGNANCY

If you are employed, a natural question to ask during pregnancy is "How long can I work?" In general, a pregnant woman is allowed to continue working until the end of pregnancy unless doing so would be hazardous to either her or her baby. The factors that need to be taken into account when you make this decision include the strenuousness of your job, the possibility of exposure to hazardous substances, your history with previous pregnancies, complications that may exist with your present pregnancy, and policies at your place of employment.

**Physical Strain.** A job that involves strenuous physical activity is potentially hazardous because of the greater risk that you may fall down or accidentally get hit in the abdomen. Either of these could injure your uterus and harm the pregnancy. If there is potential for such injury in your job, it is best to either stop working or ask for a change in assignment.

Even if your job does not generally involve strenuous activity, however, you'll need to keep an eye out for potentially hazardous situations. Since your change in shape and the added weight of your baby will put increasing strain on your back, you will need to avoid lifting and pushing heavy objects. These activities will probably not hurt your baby, but they may harm your back. Also, if it is ever necessary for you to lift an object—even if it's just a pencil—from the floor, be sure to lower yourself by bending your knees instead of bending your back.

Remember, too, that the added weight and bulk will affect your balance and mobility, so you'll need to tread carefully on stairs and newly waxed floors and you'll need to watch out for open file drawers and wobbly furniture.

The normal physical changes associated with pregnancy may also make sitting or standing all day uncomfortable. These discomforts are generally not harmful to your pregnancy, but you'll probably need to take steps to relieve them if you plan to continue working.

For example, if your work involves long periods of standing, you may experience swelling of your feet or cramps in your legs. If this occurs, support stockings may be helpful. Also, you may find it necessary to take more frequent rest periods so that you can sit down and raise your legs.

Long periods of sitting can also cause swelling in your feet. This can often be reduced by elevating your legs on a stool. If hemorrhoids have become a problem, a soft cushion on your chair may provide comfort.

Whatever your occupation, you will need adequate periods of rest, since you will fatigue much more easily. Be certain to inform your employer as soon as you know that you are pregnant so that rest periods can be worked into your schedule.

**Radiation.** Radiation of all types may be harmful to your developing baby and you must take extreme care to avoid excessive or prolonged exposure, especially during the first trimester. Dental technicians and X-ray technicians are obvious examples of women who may have prolonged radiation exposure. Many industries, however, also use X rays to detect defects in parts and equipment. Therefore, it is important that you check with your employer about the use of radiation in your workplace

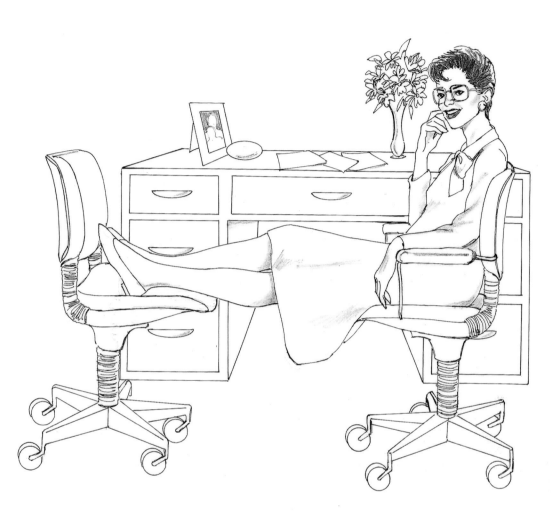

and discuss ways to avoid exposure, such as leaving the room when X rays are performed or transferring to an area in which radiation is not used. If these protective measures are not possible, you will have to stop working during your pregnancy.

Many women today work at computers with display screens for extended periods of time. To date, there is no conclusive evidence that exposure to video display terminals is harmful during pregnancy.

**Chemicals and Chemical Fumes.** Chemicals and chemical fumes are all around us; they have become a part of our modern lives. Since we deal with so many of these substances at work and at home,

we may forget that some may be potentially dangerous to the developing baby. Unfortunately, at this time, little is known about the hazardous effects of most chemicals on humans. Even less is known about the effects of certain chemicals on the unborn baby.

Therefore, as soon as you know you are pregnant, it is extremely important that you ask your employer about any chemicals that may be used in or near your work area. You should also ask about what controls and safeguards are being used for your protection. Make a list of these potential hazards (request specific names of chemicals) and discuss them with your doctor. You have the legal right

to ask your employer for this information.

Since it is impossible at this time to state that a certain chemical is absolutely safe and another is definitely harmful, it is best while you are pregnant to avoid all chemical exposure if possible. In some cases, this may mean changing your employment, while in others, it may mean wearing rubber gloves or other protective gear.

Here are some guidelines to help you avoid hazardous substances at work and at home.

- Avoid coming into contact with paints, especially those that are oil based (that includes the paint you were planning to use to paint the baby's room). Also, avoid breathing paint thinners and turpentine. It is well known that these substances will enter your body, as anyone who has ever gotten dizzy after painting knows. Scientists are not certain that these substances are harmful to the developing baby, but then again, they are not certain that they are safe. Since no one can say for sure, avoid painting products.

- If you use cleaning and polishing substances in your line of work, always wear rubber gloves when handling them and avoid splashing them onto your skin. Always work in an area with good ventilation to avoid breathing fumes. You may also want to wear a mask over your nose and mouth.
- If your job involves farming or working with plants, you may be exposed to weed killers, fertilizers, and insecticides. Some of these substances may harm your developing baby. You will probably need to change your employment if your work puts you in contact with these substances.
- Industrial plants often use dyes and substances called organic solvents during the manufacturing process. These substances are readily absorbed by the body and, in some cases, have been linked to cancer. If you have contact with these substances in your work, it is best to ask for reassignment to a safer area or quit work until after the baby is born.
- Industrial plants that make plastics also use substances such as vinyl chloride that are potentially hazardous to the developing baby. Again, if you work in such a setting, it is best to ask for a safer assignment or quit work until after you deliver your baby.
- Substances called heavy metals—lead, mercury, and others—have been associated with birth defects. Do not work with these substances during pregnancy.
- Certain gases and fumes that you may not smell or be aware of can potentially harm the baby. For example, women who work in hospital operating rooms are exposed to gases used in administering anesthetics. Women who work near running automobiles or engines in industrial plants are exposed to carbon monoxide and exhaust

---

## Certain gases may harm your baby.

---

fumes. Since little is currently known about the effects of some of these gases and fumes, it is always best to avoid them whenever possible during pregnancy.

**Infectious Organisms.** In addition to radiation and chemicals, certain infectious organisms can be harmful to your developing baby. Women who work in settings such as hospitals, laboratories, or research centers may be exposed to a variety of these potentially harmful bacteria and viruses. Since these organisms can enter your body and, in some cases, cross the placenta, the baby can become infected.

If you work in such a setting, let your employer know as soon as you suspect that you are pregnant. You will probably need to be reassigned to an area where you will not be exposed to the organisms themselves or to patients who may be infected with them.

**Complications in Prior Pregnancies.** Another factor that may influence your ability to work during pregnancy is a history of complications with previous pregnancies. Since these complications could repeat themselves in your present pregnancy, you may need to take special precautions that may conflict with your employment.

For example, if you delivered a growth-retarded baby or developed extremely high blood pressure (preeclampsia) during a previous pregnancy, your doctor may advise you to stop working and get as much rest as possible. This may also be true if you previously delivered a premature baby or if you developed serious back problems.

If it will be necessary for you to stop work early because you developed complications in a previous pregnancy, your doctor should be able to inform you of this at your first office visit. If so, it is best to let your employer know as soon as possible.

**Complications in Current Pregnancy.** Certain problems or complications in your present pregnancy may also force you to stop work early. Women who are carrying more than one baby are generally advised to stop working during their seventh or eighth month. If you have experienced abnormal bleeding or premature labor contractions, or if you have high blood pressure or diabetes, your doctor may also advise you to stop work early.

**Policies at Work.** Before you become pregnant, it is probably best to check with your employer about policies regarding pregnancy. For example, check on your insurance coverage for maternity care and the length of time that you can take off from work both before and after delivery of your baby.

There are now laws that protect pregnant women from discrimination in employment. In general, employers are required by law to treat pregnancy and childbirth as they do any other physical disability. The "Pregnancy Discrimination Act," which went into effect in 1979, prohibits employers from discriminating against women on the basis of pregnancy, childbirth, and related conditions. To avoid any problems, it is always best to notify your employer as soon as possible about your intention to stop working or about your need for reassignment to a safer area.

## TRAVELING FOR TWO

Another question that you may ask when you are pregnant is "How far and how long can I safely travel?" Since each pregnancy is unique, it is difficult to establish one policy that would apply to all pregnant women. There are, however, some basic guidelines that do apply to most pregnancies.

In general, if your pregnancy has been normal, there is no physical reason why you should not travel. However, since an emergency can occur at any time, it is always best to avoid remote destinations where medical facilities and competent obstetrical care may not be available.

During your last month of pregnancy, when labor is most likely, most doctors advise that you travel no farther than one hour's distance away from the hospital where you plan to deliver.

If you are experiencing any complications with your current pregnancy, you should discuss any travel plans with your doctor. If you do have permission to travel, it's wise to bring along a list of medical facilities at your destination in case you experience any problems.

**Traveling by Car.** Whenever you travel in an automobile, be sure to wear a seat belt with a shoulder restraint. The lap belt should be placed snugly across your hips *below* the bulge of your abdomen. The shoulder belt should be placed *above* your abdomen and between your breasts. Never wear a seat belt across your abdomen.

Ask your doctor if it is all right for you to drive a car yourself. In most cases, if your pregnancy has been normal, this will be permitted. During your last month of pregnancy, however, you'll probably need to give up the driver's seat,

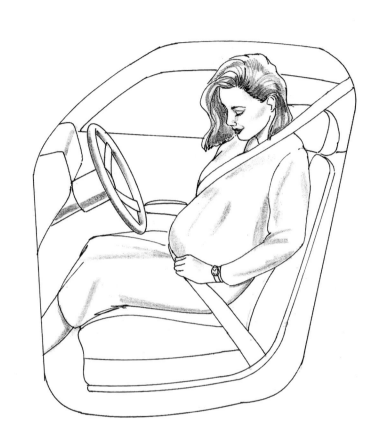

since your large abdomen may make controlling the steering wheel difficult.

When traveling long distances by automobile, it is important to make frequent rest stops—at least once every hour—to change position, stretch your legs, and use the rest room. Since it will usually not be possible to elevate your legs during a car trip, you may wish to wear support stockings to prevent your feet from swelling. In addition, since long car trips are fatiguing, even to those who are not pregnant, you may wish to get extra sleep the night before your trip.

**Traveling by Air.** In some cases, it may be preferable or necessary to travel by airplane, since the time needed to get to your destination will be shorter. To make your trip more comfortable, try to

get a seat on the aisle. This way, you won't have to climb over other people each time you need to use the rest room. Be sure to wear your seat belt snugly across your hips below your abdomen whenever you are seated. You may also want to wear support hose to keep your feet from swelling and place a pillow behind the small of your back to make sitting more comfortable.

During your last few months of pregnancy, most airlines will ask to see a letter from your doctor that indicates your due date and states that you are in good health and able to travel. Remember, too, that during your last month of pregnancy, your doctor will probably recommend that you travel no farther than one hour's distance from the hospital in which you intend to deliver.

# Pregnancy After 35

The woman who delayed pregnancy until she was in her 30s or 40s was the exception years ago. Today, however, it is increasingly common for a woman to bear her first child when she is in the third or fourth decade of her life. Career plans, pursuit of education, improved health care, and more reliable forms of contraception are but a few of the factors contributing to the trend of delayed childbearing.

By medical tradition, an "older" mother is defined as a woman who becomes pregnant when she is 35 years of age or older. Today, however, authorities agree that there is no reason for a woman over the age of 35 who has not reached menopause to give up the idea of pregnancy merely by reason of her age.

Although most pregnant women over the age of 35 will experience successful pregnancies and deliver healthy babies, there are some problems that are more likely to occur in the older mother.

**Infertility.** The inability to become pregnant—called infertility—is more common among older women. Because women begin to ovulate (produce eggs) less frequently at about age 30, the number of opportunities to achieve fertilization decreases as each year goes by. For example, the average healthy woman at age 30 will ovulate 13 times a year; by the time she has reached 40, she may ovulate only five or six times a year.

Older women are also more likely to have problems with their reproductive organs that may prevent pregnancy. Extensive endometriosis (a condition in which endometrial tissue from the lining of the uterus becomes detached and grows in the abdominal cavity outside the uterus) and uterine fibroids (solid, noncancerous tumors that grow within the walls of the uterus or outward from the uterine wall) may make it difficult or impossible to become pregnant.

**Chronic Illness.** As we grow older, we are more likely to develop chronic illnesses, such as high blood pressure, diabetes, and glandular disorders like hypothyroidism (underactive thyroid gland). Although these illnesses can usually be controlled fairly easily in the nonpregnant woman, they may become more serious or even uncontrollable during pregnancy and thus threaten the well-being of both mother and baby. What's more, certain chronic illnesses of the mother are associated with an increased risk of miscarriage and stillbirth.

For these reasons, doctors suggest that if you are over the age of 35 and wish to become pregnant, it is best to get a thorough medical checkup before you attempt to conceive. If certain chronic illnesses are detected, they can be completely evaluated and brought under control before pregnancy.

If you are over 35 and are currently pregnant, be sure to discuss with your doctor any chronic illnesses you may have. Your condition will be monitored more closely during pregnancy, and special precautions, such as bed rest, can be taken to help prevent further complications (see *Special Situations*, p. 76, for more on chronic illness in pregnancy).

**Birth Defects.** Older mothers are also at greater risk of having babies with severe birth defects caused by abnormalities in the baby's chromosomes.

Chromosomes are structures contained within all cells of the body, including the egg and the sperm. These chromosomes contain the genetic information that is passed on from parents to baby. Normally, the sperm and the egg each contain 23 chromosomes. When the sperm and the egg join, the resulting cell, which will develop to form the baby, will contain the normal chromosome number of 46.

In some cases, however, the resulting fertilized egg contains 47 chromosomes—an abnormal number. The baby that results will then have 47 chromosomes in most or all of the cells in her body.

In many cases, a fetus with an abnormal chromosome number will miscarry, accounting somewhat for the higher miscarriage rate in older women. In those pregnancies that continue, the fetus will usually be born with any one of a number of physical or mental abnormalities.

The most common condition associated with an abnormal chromosome number is Down's syndrome. Babies born with this condition are mentally retarded and may have serious abnormalities of the heart and digestive system. Children with Down's syndrome have a characteristic facial appearance marked by slanted eyes, heavy eyebrows, and a large, thick tongue.

Although Down's syndrome can occur in babies born to mothers of any age, it occurs more frequently in babies born to older mothers. At the age of 20, a mother has one chance in 1,667 of having a child with Down's syndrome; at the age of 35, she has one chance in 370; at age 40, she has one chance in 109.

Although the father's age may have some effect on risk, it is much less significant than the effect of the mother's age. If you have any questions about the effect your age or your husband's age may have on your baby, be sure to discuss them with your doctor.

**Complications in Pregnancy, Labor, or Delivery.** During pregnancy, the older mother may experience more aches and pains, such as backache and leg pain, due to "aging" of her bones and muscles.

Beyond these minor discomforts, however, the older woman is at a somewhat higher risk of developing certain potentially serious complications. An older woman, for example, is more likely than a younger woman to develop severely elevated blood pressure (preeclampsia) during pregnancy.

Placental abruption, in which the placenta becomes detached from the uterine wall before the baby is born, is also more common among older mothers. Placental abruption can lead to severe bleeding in the mother and oxygen deprivation in the baby.

For unknown reasons, the older mother is also more likely to have twins.

Most older mothers experience a normal labor and delivery. Because certain complications are more common among older women, however, the rate of cesarean section is somewhat higher in older mothers.

Even though pregnancy in older women is associated with an increase in certain complications, it's important to keep in mind that the majority of older mothers deliver healthy babies. As in any pregnancy, good prenatal care can help the older mother decrease her risk of experiencing complications and greatly increase the chances that her baby will be born healthy.

## Prenatal Care for the Older Mother

The prenatal care of an older mother is generally like that of a woman in any other age group. It involves proper diet and weight gain, adequate exercise and rest, and careful monitoring through prenatal visits. If the mother has a history of high blood pressure, diabetes, or other chronic disorders, prenatal office visits may be more frequent than usual, especially during the last two months of pregnancy.

In addition to this basic prenatal care, mothers 35 years of age and older will be offered amniocentesis—a test to determine the presence of chromosome abnormalities in the baby. This test is performed between the sixteenth and eighteenth weeks of pregnancy.

Immediately before performing an amniocentesis, an ultrasound study (see p.48) is performed to determine the exact location of both the baby and the placenta. After an area of skin on the mother's abdomen has been anesthetized, the doctor inserts a long, hollow needle through the mother's abdominal wall and into the uterus (the ultrasound study helps the doctor to insert the needle without harming the baby). With the needle in the amniotic sac surrounding the baby, the doctor draws about two tablespoons of amniotic fluid into a syringe. This fluid contains cells that have fallen off the skin of the baby. After these cells have been grown on a special culture plate and examined under a microscope, the chromosomes of the baby are analyzed to see if there is an abnormal number.

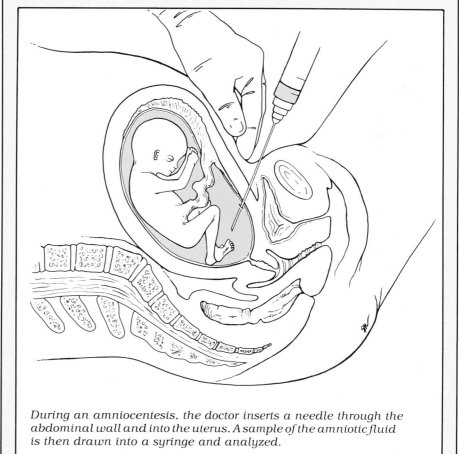

*During an amniocentesis, the doctor inserts a needle through the abdominal wall and into the uterus. A sample of the amniotic fluid is then drawn into a syringe and analyzed.*

# THE
# SECOND
# TRIMESTER

The physical changes that occur during pregnancy, both in the baby and in you, are dramatic and wondrous. Two tiny cells join together within your body and, from that union, an entirely new person is created.

The many complex organs and structures that your baby will need for life develop in just a few short months. The changes in your body are no less amazing. But while the baby changes most rapidly during the first three months after conception, your body undergoes its most dramatic changes during your second and third trimesters.

It is during your second trimester that your baby will announce his presence. Early in this trimester, you will actually begin to see and feel your abdomen enlarging in response to his growth. What's more, you and your husband will be able to feel your baby's movements through the wall of your abdomen.

While many of the discomforts you experienced in your first trimester have probably begun to subside, the next three months will bring a host of new changes. Many of these changes will occur in response to your growing abdomen—and your growing baby.

In the following sections, you'll discover what's going on inside the womb, how your body is changing, how to tell if something is wrong, and how to avoid hazards. You'll find tips for relieving the discomforts that accompany the changes in your size and shape. You'll also find information on exercise and childbirth classes. This information, coupled with your attention to good nutrition, can help you take good care of yourself and your growing baby.

# Your Growing Baby

By his fourth month, your baby's organs are completely developed and are beginning to function, but not yet to the point where he can live outside your body. This month marks the start of a period of very rapid growth as well as the formation of some finishing touches on the face and body that will give your baby a clearly human appearance.

From head to toe, your baby is now about seven inches long and weighs about four ounces. Lanugo—a fine, downy growth of hair—appears on the skin all over his body. (This coat of hair will fall out before birth.) Eyebrows, eyelashes, and scalp hairs also begin to grow. In those babies destined to have dark hair, pigment cells in the hair follicles start making the dark pigment that will give the hair its color.

Also during this month, the baby's face develops further and becomes more "babylike." His chin is still small compared to the rest of his head, and his eyes are quite large and widely spaced. But during the next two months, his

### Your baby is now very active.

face will grow rapidly, and at birth his eyes and chin will look just right.

Also during this month, the baby's mouth, tongue, and throat continue to form. Vocal cords and taste buds have now developed, even though they will not be used for several months to come.

By the end of his fourth month, your baby has become larger and stronger. His muscles are growing, his newly forming bones are getting longer, and his body is becoming more solid. It is about this time that you may actually begin to feel the baby move. At first, you may only feel a slight flutter that may make you think that you have indigestion or gas. But by the time you are in your fifth month, you will easily recognize the kicks that announce your baby.

Even though you may not always feel him, your baby is now extremely active—moving his arms and legs, making breathing movements, twisting his body, and swallowing amniotic fluid. Most of the time, he is probably moving to get into a more comfortable position, but at other times, he may be reacting to your movement and even to sounds inside and outside your body. You may also find that your baby becomes more active shortly after you eat. This is easy to understand, since the baby just got an energy boost from your body.

The placenta, too, has grown rapidly. By the fourth month, the yolk sac has disappeared and your baby is obtaining all of his nourishment through the placenta. The baby's heart pumps his blood through the blood vessels in the umbilical cord to reach the placenta. Once in the placenta, oxygen, minerals, and other nutrients pass from your blood to your baby's blood. Your blood and your baby's blood, however, don't actually mix. Rather, they pass close to each other, separated by a thin membrane that allows certain substances to pass. Your baby's blood then circulates back to your baby through the umbilical cord. The umbilical cord also carries certain waste products from your baby back to the placenta so that these wastes may be transferred to your blood and excreted from your body.

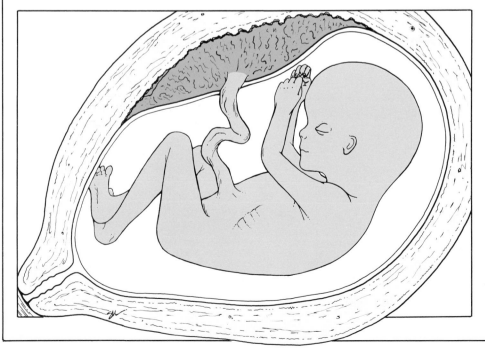

# MONTH

# Your Changing Body

Now that you have reached the fourth month of pregnancy, most of the discomforts that you felt during the first trimester have probably subsided. Morning sickness is less severe, urination is practically back to normal, and you have a renewed feeling of energy. The baby will soon be giving you little kicks to remind you that he is there, and chances are, you will generally feel good all over.

This month, something new and exciting occurs—you can actually begin to see and feel your enlarging uterus. Lie down perfectly flat, relax your abdominal muscles, and feel the firm, smooth bulge above the bone that lies beneath your pubic hair. You are now beginning to "show."

Even though you are probably very happy about being pregnant, you may also become somewhat self-conscious or even embarrassed about your change in shape. Don't worry; proper exercise can help you return to your prepregnancy appearance within a few months after delivery.

At about this time in pregnancy, you will probably begin to develop backache. This rather annoying problem is experienced by nearly every pregnant woman and tends to be worse with a second pregnancy compared to the first.

Backache occurs because your body is attempting to adapt to your new shape and to the extra weight that you are now carrying in your abdomen. If you notice other pregnant women, especially those very near delivery, you will see that they tend to walk and stand with their backs arched backward. This is the body's way of compensating for a protruding abdomen. This arching, however, puts a constant

strain on the back muscles and causes them to ache. The hormone progesterone also relaxes some of the supporting tissues in your back and adds to the development of backache.

By now, you may also have noticed that you have developed cravings for certain foods or other substances. Some women have cravings that are quite unusual

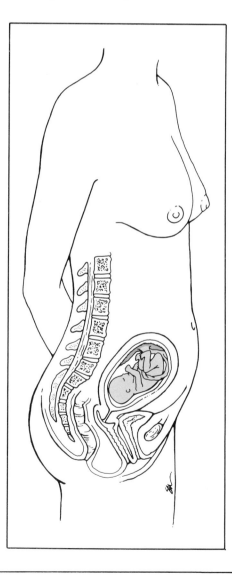

and may include laundry starch, clay, and even the frosty ice that forms inside of freezers. No one

---

## This month, you will begin to see and feel your abdomen growing.

---

knows exactly why cravings develop, but in some cases it is believed to occur when there is a lack of certain nutrients in the diet.

Cravings are extremely common and normally will harm neither you nor your baby. If you have questions about foods or other substances that you might crave, it is always best to ask your doctor.

There are several skin changes that commonly occur at this point in pregnancy, and they are all caused by your increasing levels of hormones. Palmar erythema is a term that refers to the reddening of the palms of the hands that commonly begins in the second trimester. This reddening is not abnormal; rather, it is caused by an increase in the amount of blood flowing through the hands. Spider nevi are another common skin change. These appear as tiny broken blood vessels, usually on the skin over the abdomen and chest. These skin changes will disappear after delivery of the baby.

You may also notice an increase in perspiration and in the oiliness of your skin. In some cases, you may actually develop a mild case of acne because of this excess oil. These changes also disappear after delivery.

# Do I Need Special Tests?

## Three medical tests, now commonly performed during pregnancy, can greatly increase the safety of both the mother and the baby.

The tremendous advances made in obstetrics over the last two decades have greatly increased the safety of both mother and baby during pregnancy. Among these advances are three common tests that can help determine the health of your baby while he is still in your uterus.

**Ultrasound.** This is one of the most commonly used tests in obstetrics today. An ultrasound test involves the use of a machine that sends sound waves through your abdominal wall and uterus. These sound waves rebound off the baby's tissue and the placenta and are transmitted back to a screen to

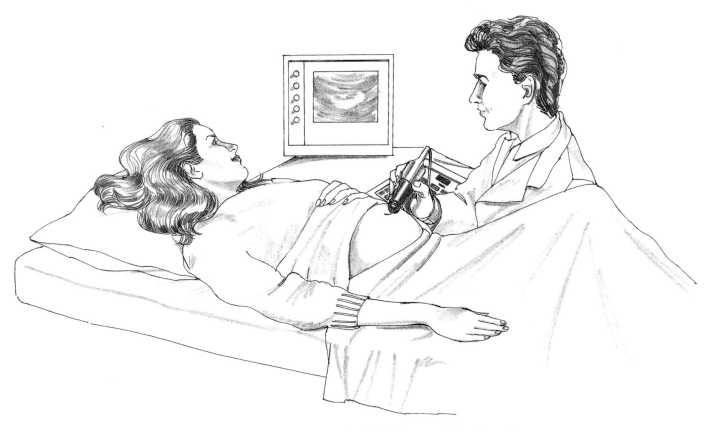

*An ultrasound study uses sound waves to create a "picture" of the baby and the placenta.*

form a "picture" of the baby and placenta. Using ultrasound, your doctor can "see" inside your uterus and gain valuable information about the development of the baby and the placenta.

An ultrasound test is most commonly performed during pregnancy for one or more of the following reasons.

- To determine the age of the baby if there is a question about the dates of your last menstrual period
- To check the size of the baby to make sure he is growing normally
- To determine the location of the placenta if you experience vaginal bleeding
- To determine if you are carrying more than one baby
- To detect physical abnormalities in the baby or placenta
- To determine the location of the baby and placenta before amniocentesis
- To locate the site of the pregnancy if it is suspected to be outside the uterus (ectopic pregnancy)

The entire ultrasound procedure takes about 15 to 20 minutes and causes no discomfort. To date, no harmful effects of ultrasound have been found for either mother or baby.

**Alpha-fetoprotein (AFP) Screening.** Alpha-fetoprotein is a substance, produced by the developing baby, that passes into the mother's bloodstream through the umbilical cord. Normally, only a small amount of alpha-fetoprotein enters the mother's blood. However, in cases where the baby suffers from a neural tube defect, such as spina bifida (failure of the spinal column to close completely) or anencephaly (failure of the brain to develop), alpha-fetoprotein levels in the mother's blood are abnormally high.

Neural tube defects occur approximately once in every thousand births. Since these defects are so common, testing for alpha-fetoprotein is now recommended for all pregnant women.

The test is best performed about 16 to 18 weeks after the first day of your last menstrual period

---

## Ask your doctor about these tests.

---

and involves taking a small sample of your blood. Results are usually available in less than one week.

**Amniocentesis.** This procedure involves the removal of a small amount of amniotic fluid from the amniotic sac that surrounds the baby. The fluid is obtained by inserting a needle through the walls of your abdomen and uterus.

Before an amniocentesis is performed, an ultrasound test is done to determine the exact location of the baby and the placenta. Next, the skin over your abdomen is cleansed and a small amount of local anesthetic is injected to numb the skin. Using the ultrasound picture as a guide, the doctor inserts a hollow needle through the skin and into the uterus. About two tablespoons of amniotic fluid are then extracted with a syringe.

A laboratory analysis of the amniotic fluid can provide your doctor with information about the baby's health. For example, the fluid itself can be analyzed to determine if the baby has Tay-Sachs disease or other serious inherited conditions. The fluid can also be analyzed for the presence of surfactant, a substance that develops in the baby's lungs during the third trimester to prevent his lungs from collapsing at birth. This analysis can help your doctor to determine if the baby will be able to breathe normally outside your body.

Cells that have been shed from the baby's skin are also present in the amniotic fluid and can be cultured and analyzed to determine if the baby has any chromosome abnormalities such as Down's syndrome.

The discomforts of amniocentesis are minor, but the test does involve some risk of infection and other complications. Therefore, an amniocentesis should be performed only after you and your doctor have determined that the possible benefits of the test outweigh the possible risks. If the test is necessary, it will be performed between the sixteenth and eighteenth week after the first day of your last menstrual period.

---

## This Month's Visit

During this month's office visit, the doctor will probably:

- Check your weight. By now, you will have gained about six to eight pounds.
- Check your blood pressure. Your blood pressure may now be slightly below what it was before pregnancy.
- Check your urine for sugar and protein. You should normally have neither sugar nor protein in your urine.
- Ask about symptoms of pregnancy. You may now be experiencing backache.
- Ask how you are feeling.
- Ask if you can feel the baby moving. You may begin to feel movement toward the end of this month.
- Check the growth of the uterus by feeling your lower abdomen. By the end of this month, the top of the uterus will be about halfway between your pubic bone and your navel.
- Listen for the baby's heartbeat. You and your doctor will easily hear the heartbeat by using an instrument called a doppler.
- Perform a blood test for alpha-fetoprotein (see this month's *Ask the Doctor*).

# Safe Exercise and Activity

Proper exercise during pregnancy can provide you with a host of benefits. It can improve your muscle tone and strength, which will help you adjust to your increasing weight and changing posture. It can help improve the circulation of blood in your arms and legs and help you deal with some of the minor discomforts of pregnancy. It can prepare your body for labor and delivery by increasing your flexibility and strength. It can improve your self-image and sense of well-being. And it can make getting back into shape after delivery easier.

Fortunately, you don't have to train like an Olympic athlete to achieve these benefits. Rather, you can choose and follow a regular pattern of exercise and activity that suits both your pregnancy and your lifestyle.

## WHERE TO BEGIN

Becoming physically fit and maintaining that fitness during pregnancy requires engaging regularly in safe, moderate, and sustained exercise. Of course, pregnancy is not the time to embark on a rigorous new sport or engage in strenuous workouts. On the other hand, even if you have never exercised regularly before, you can safely begin a workout program during pregnancy (see the *Exercising Caution* section for exceptions).

**The First-Time Exerciser.** Women who have not exercised regularly before pregnancy are encouraged to begin a program of moderate exercise as soon as possible. If you're beginning your program late in your pregnancy, however, you may need to choose

your activity more carefully and start out more slowly because of alterations that may have already taken place in your ligaments and muscles. Discuss with your doctor the appropriate type of exercise for each stage of pregnancy.

The safest and most productive activities during pregnancy, especially for the woman exercising for the first time, are swimming and brisk walking. They are best because they can usually be continued until almost the day of delivery and because they carry little risk of injury that would harm the pregnancy or prevent further exercising. All you need before beginning is a sound program, appropriate clothing, and a health clearance from your doctor.

**Continuing Your Current Program.** Women who were engaged in an exercise program before pregnancy are usually encouraged to continue during pregnancy, as long as the activity does not involve much risk of falls or other injuries. In general, sports that carry a high risk of falling or getting hit—for example, skiing, skating, horseback riding, basketball—are not recommended. Discuss your current exercise plan with your doctor; she will tell you if there are any restrictions that she wants to place on your activities.

You may find that you need to modify or slow the pace of your usual exercise program due to fatigue in early pregnancy or due to added weight and the normal softening of joint ligaments in late pregnancy. Your body is your best guide and usually responds with pain or fatigue if an activity becomes inappropriate.

**Exercising Caution.** No single exercise program is suitable for all

pregnant women. In some cases, exercise will be modified or even prohibited if the woman has certain medical conditions, complications with the current pregnancy, or a history of complications with a previous pregnancy. It is particularly important that you not begin exercising without your doctor's approval if:

- You have any type of heart or lung condition.
- You have diabetes that developed before or during pregnancy.
- You have high blood pressure.
- You have a history of premature labor.
- Your placenta is implanted completely over or near your cervix (placenta previa).
- You have physical impairments or diseases of the muscles or bones.
- You have had more than three miscarriages.
- You have experienced cramping, spotting, or bleeding during this pregnancy.
- You are carrying more than one baby.

Should any of these conditions apply to you, consult your doctor and follow her guidelines.

**Guidelines for Safe Exercise.** In addition to your doctor's advice, the following general guidelines can help make exercise during pregnancy safe and enjoyable.

*Exercise regularly.* Plan ahead and give yourself specific times during the day to dedicate to exercise. You can't make up for lost time, so don't push yourself too hard to catch up. Instead, make exercise a habit from the start.

*Stop if you feel pain.* Modify your exercise program if necessary or substitute other forms of exercise. If pain persists or is severe, check with your doctor immediately.

*Finish eating at least one hour before exercising.* Exercising too soon after a meal can cause burping and abdominal discomfort.

*Drink water before, during, and after a workout.* You will need to keep adequate amounts of fluids in your body to prevent fatigue. Also, during pregnancy you may be more likely to faint if you are dehydrated. Exactly how much fluid you will need depends on the climate you are in and the type of exercise you are doing. In general, you will need to drink at least one extra glass of water for every hour that you exercise.

*Maintain adequate nutrition.* When you are pregnant, you are advised to add 300 extra calories to your daily diet. If you exercise in addition to performing your everyday activities during pregnancy, you will need even more. In general, you may need as many as 150 to 300 additional calories for each hour that you exercise.

*Don't get overheated.* Avoid exercising in a hot room and avoid exercising outdoors if the temperature is above 90 degrees Fahrenheit.

*Stop exercising if you develop symptoms of overexertion.* These include nausea, vomiting, headache, light-headedness, dizziness, extreme shortness of breath, tightness in the chest, and extreme perspiration. If any of these symptoms occurs, stop exercising immediately and call your doctor.

*Exercise gently and respect your body.* Always warm up slowly and avoid strain (see *Your Workout Routine*).

*Limit the amount of time that you spend lying flat on your back.* In this position, the heavy uterus is pressing down on the major blood vessels within your abdomen that return blood to your heart.

Avoid exercises and activities that require you to lie on your back for more than five minutes at a time, especially during the third trimester.

*Avoid exercises that put a strain on your lower back, hips, or pelvic joints.* Among the exercises to avoid are double leg raises, full sit-ups, and any exercise that requires you to arch your back inward.

---

## Be sure to check with your doctor *before* beginning an exercise program during pregnancy.

---

*Sit up and lie down slowly.* This is important in order to avoid straining your back. When raising or lowering your body, roll over to one side and use your arms and legs to do the work.

*Avoid exercises and dance movements that require good balance and quick moves.* Your changing size and shape will make such refined movements difficult and will increase your chance of falling.

*Avoid jumping, hopping, skipping, and bouncing.* Bouncing while stretching does not effectively condition muscles and can lead to back injury. Exercises that involve a lot of jumping, hopping, and skipping put a strain on the joints and increase the likelihood of falls.

*Avoid raising both legs off the floor at the same time.* This, too, may strain the lower back muscles.

*Exercise on a supportive surface.* Avoid lying on flat, hard surfaces. To better cushion your body, always exercise on either grass, carpet, or a foam mat.

*Do not remain at peak exercise capacity for longer than*

15 minutes without being supervised. It is not advisable for your heart rate to exceed about 120 beats per minute for long periods of time.

*Check with your doctor before starting any exercise program.* Your doctor can advise you about the type, intensity, and duration of exercise that is appropriate at various stages of pregnancy.

*Have fun when you exercise.* A well-planned exercise program should be enjoyable and should promote a sense of well-being. Exercise at a pace that is comfortable for you.

**Clothing.** When you exercise, it is also important that you wear appropriate clothing, not only for comfort, but also for safety. The following are general guidelines.

*Wear loose-fitting, comfortable clothes that allow perspiration to evaporate.* Comfort is more important than glamour.

*Wear a good support bra while exercising.* In pregnancy, your breasts are larger, and the supporting tissues may be somewhat relaxed due to hormonal influences. For exercising, an adequate bra should provide firm support and limit bouncing. It should be sturdy and nonchafing and should fit well, especially around the edges of the breasts beneath the arms. "Sports bras" that meet all of these requirements are available in large sporting-goods and department stores.

If your breasts are very large and heavy, wear two bras for extra support and comfort during your workout. Wearing a nursing/maternity bra beneath a sports bra (or vice versa if that's more comfortable) works very nicely to minimize bouncing and increase comfort.

*Wear good shoes.* Walking and aerobic dancing involve contact with relatively hard surfaces. Proper shoes provide protection, support, cushioning, traction, and flexibility. What you will need is a good pair of walking shoes or aerobic shoes with adequate arch supports, heel cushioning, and lateral (side) support. They're generally available in sporting-goods stores.

## PRENATAL EXERCISES

Exercises that you perform during pregnancy can be conveniently divided into prenatal exercises, which are intended to maintain general physical fitness and well-being, and childbirth exercises, which are intended to provide you with strength, coordination, and control of the muscles that you will use during labor and delivery.

When choosing a prenatal exercise program to build and maintain physical fitness, you'll want to find an activity that provides your body with a good aerobic workout.

**What's an Aerobic Exercise?** An activity or exercise is aerobic if it creates an increased need for oxygen over a sustained period. In other words, it should make your heart work harder and make you breathe more deeply and rapidly than usual over an extended period of time. Examples of aerobic exercise include lap swimming, brisk walking, jogging, biking, rowing, dancing, and cross-country skiing.

**Benefits of Aerobic Exercise.** Engaging in regular aerobic exercise during pregnancy can provide a variety of health benefits. Aerobic exercise can:

- Strengthen and tone the walls of your blood vessels, which enhances circulation.
- Increase your lung capacity, providing more oxygen for the uterus, the placenta, and the baby.
- Increase your stamina and endurance, enabling you to do more without tiring as quickly. This will be especially important to you during the strenuous process of labor and delivery.

- Help make recovery after delivery easier, since physically fit women generally recover more quickly.

---

## Spend at least ten minutes stretching and warming up before each aerobic workout.

---

**Choosing a Safe Aerobic Exercise.** Many popular recreational activities qualify not only as good aerobic workouts but also as safe prenatal exercise. For example, lap swimming is one of the best activities that pregnant women can do to safely develop strength, coordination, and aerobic fitness. It's also easy on the joints. All of the standard strokes are safe to use. If you decide to swim for exercise, always remember to swim in an uncrowded area to avoid being kicked or bumped.

Brisk walking, too, provides excellent exercise for the pregnant woman. You'll need to choose an area where you are unlikely to trip and fall and where you will not have to overexert yourself on steep hills. You'll also need to walk at a pace that's quick enough to get your heart pumping faster without being uncomfortable. A good guide to follow is the "talk test." You should be moving at a pace that makes you breathe more rapidly, but you should still be able to hold a conversation as you walk. If you can't, slow down. Discuss with your doctor the pace and duration of exercise that's right for you at each stage of pregnancy.

If you jogged before pregnancy, you may be able to continue, but you should limit yourself to less than two miles a day. It's best to discuss this with your doctor. If you were not an active jogger before

pregnancy, now is not the time to take up the sport.

You may also be able to find a specially designed prenatal aerobics class in your area. Aerobics, however, are not recommended during pregnancy except under a supervised program that has been approved by your doctor.

**Your Workout Routine.** No matter which aerobic activity you choose for maintaining your physical fitness during pregnancy, each of your workouts or exercise sessions should consist of three parts: a warm-up period, an aerobic workout, and a cool-down period.

*The warm-up.* No aerobic workout should be started with a "cold" body. Warm-up moves tell your body that more vigorous activity is coming and help prevent injury by releasing muscle tension and making the body more flexible.

Spend at least five to ten minutes stretching and limbering up before each workout. (You'll find three simple stretches in the section that follows.) Stretch just to the point of mild tension (not pain) and then hold the stretch for a slow count of ten. Don't bounce; it will only make your muscles tighter. Release and repeat each stretch three times in all.

Concentrate your stretching mainly on the lower body (legs, ankles, hips, knees), but don't completely neglect the upper body (arms, shoulders, neck).

Once you've stretched adequately, spend five more minutes moving slowly (for example, walk slowly or do a few leisurely strokes in the pool) before increasing your pace.

*The aerobic workout.* Before beginning your aerobic exercise program, ask your doctor about an acceptable heart rate that can be sustained during your workouts.

Once you have stretched your muscles and warmed up your body for your workout, you can gradually increase your pace until you've reached the target heart rate recommended by your doctor. Spend 12 to 15 minutes exercising at this level.

*The cool-down.* Once you complete your workout, slow down your activity gradually over a five-minute period. Stretch again for five to ten minutes.

**Stretches to Get You Started.** Here are three stretches that you can use to limber up the muscles in your back and legs. They're especially useful to do as part of the warm-up and cool-down for your aerobic workout. Hold each stretch for ten seconds.

### Calf Stretch

1. Face a wall. Stand a short distance from the wall and rest your forearms on the wall. Place your forehead on the backs of your hands and keep your back straight.
2. Bend one knee and bring it toward the wall. Keep the back leg straight and the back foot flat on the floor.
3. Create an easy feeling of stretch in your calf muscle, hold for ten seconds, then release.

### Deep Calf and Achilles Tendon Stretch

1. Start in the same position described in the first step of the Calf Stretch.
2. Bend one knee and bring it toward the wall.
3. Lower your hips as you bend your other knee slightly. Be sure to keep your back straight and your feet flat on the floor. Your back foot should point either straight ahead or slightly inward during the stretch.
4. Hold this stretch for ten seconds, then release.

### Back, Calf, and Hamstring Stretch

1. Sit on the floor with one leg stretched straight out in front of you; the back of the knee should be flat on the floor. Rest the other leg on the floor with the knee bent and out to the side.
2. Stretch easily, then lean forward from the hips to increase the stretch.
3. Hold for ten seconds, then release.

*Calf Stretch*
*(Step 2)*

*Deep Calf and Tendon Stretch*
*(Step 3)*

*Back, Calf, and Hamstring*
*Stretch (Step 2)*

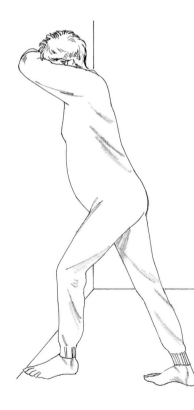

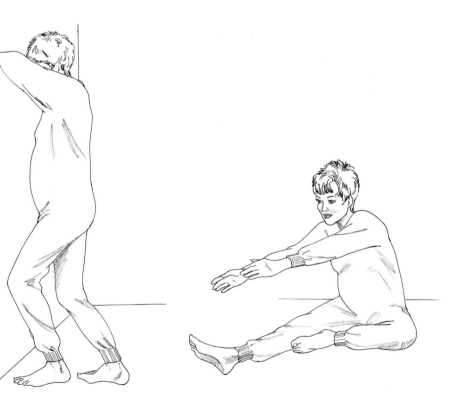

## CHILDBIRTH EXERCISES

In addition to participating in regular prenatal aerobic exercise, you can also engage in exercises designed specifically to prepare your body for labor and delivery. These so-called childbirth exercises, when performed regularly throughout pregnancy, can help you strengthen your abdominal muscles, improve your coordination and flexibility, and relax the muscles that are important in both labor and delivery.

### Pelvic Tilt

The purpose of this exercise is to strengthen the abdominal muscles and stretch the lower back.
1. Get down on your hands and knees on the floor. Your hands should be directly below your shoulders and your legs should be directly below your hips. Be sure to keep your back straight; never let your back sag downward.
2. Exhale as you tighten your abdominal muscles and buttocks and press up with your lower back.
3. Hold this position for three seconds. Inhale and relax. Repeat five times.

### Variation

1. Lie on your back with your knees bent and your feet flat on the floor.
2. Exhale as you tilt your pelvis back by pulling in your abdomen and pushing the lower part of your back against the floor.
3. Hold this position for a slow count of six. Then inhale and relax, allowing your back to return to the resting position. Repeat this ten times.

### Leg Raising

The purpose of this exercise is to increase abdominal and leg strength and coordinate breathing with muscular activity.
1. Lie on your back, then bend one knee and place your foot flat on the floor. Keep your other leg straight.
2. Exhale as you push the lower part of your back against the floor and pull in your abdomen (as in the variation of the Pelvic Tilt).
3. Inhale and raise your straight leg up toward the ceiling; do not point your toes.
4. Lower your leg slowly while exhaling through your mouth. Make certain that you maintain the pelvic tilt throughout the entire exercise. Repeat the exercise raising the opposite leg. Repeat five times for each leg.

*Pelvic Tilt
(Step 1)*

*Leg Raising
(Step 3)*

*Pelvic Tilt
(Step 2)*

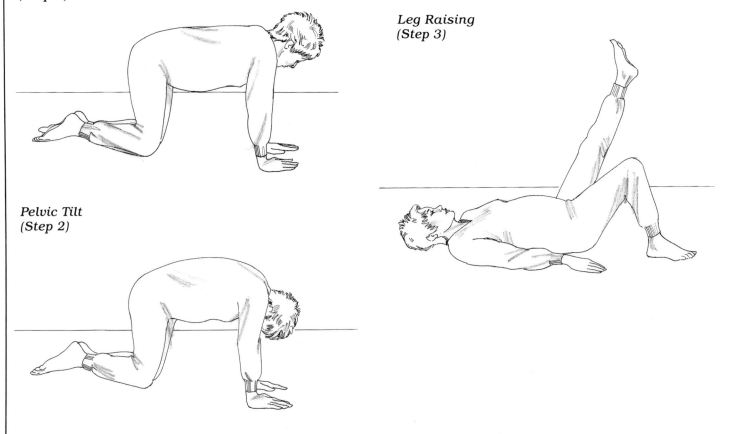

## Curl-Up

The purpose of this exercise is to strengthen your abdomen.

1. Lie on your back with your pelvis tilted, your knees bent, and your feet flat on the floor.

2. Stretch your hands toward your knees and raise your head and shoulders off the floor as you breathe out through your mouth.

3. Slowly relax, breathe in, and resume your starting position. Repeat five times.

## Bridging

The purpose of this exercise is to strengthen your hip muscles and maintain flexibility.

1. Lie on your back with your knees bent and your feet flat on the floor.

2. Lift your hips off the floor while keeping your back straight.

3. Hold for three seconds, then relax and resume your starting position. Repeat five times.

## Pelvic Floor Contraction (Kegel Exercise)

During pregnancy, the weight of the baby and the uterus strains the muscles of the pelvis. Furthermore, during delivery, these muscles are stretched even more as the baby passes into the vagina. Since these same muscles are important for keeping your bladder and reproductive organs in their proper positions, specific exercises should be performed during pregnancy to preserve their strength and tone.

These exercises will also increase your awareness of your pelvic muscles so that you can consciously relax them during delivery of the baby.

1. Sit, stand, or lie down comfortably.

2. Think about your vagina and anal area and tighten these muscles in the same way that you would to stop urination midstream.

3. Hold as tightly as possible for a slow count of five while breathing normally. Relax completely, then repeat. Once you have an awareness of these muscles, Kegel exercises can be done anytime and anywhere. You should try to do at least a few repetitions every day throughout pregnancy.

*Curl-Up*
*(Step 2)*

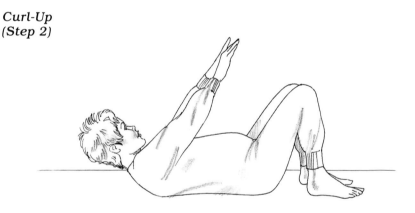

*Bridging*
*(Step 2)*

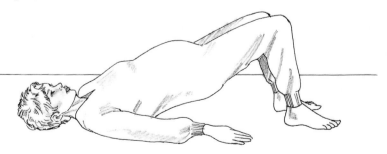

# Your Growing Baby

During the fifth month after conception, your baby continues his rapid rate of growth, and by the end of the month, he will be nearly ten inches long and will weigh ten to 12 ounces. His body is now gaining bulk, length, and considerable physical strength.

Your baby's heart has, by this time, grown to the point where your doctor can hear the heartbeat by placing a stethoscope on the skin over your uterus. The heartbeat is still quite faint, but the doctor can easily count about 140 to 150 beats per minute—a normal heartbeat for a baby at this stage of development.

On the outside, the baby is fully covered by lanugo hair and has distinct eyelashes and eyebrows. His face is becoming more babylike as his chin and facial bones continue to grow.

It is also during this month that the baby's body elongates; the length of his torso and legs rapidly increases in proportion to the size of his head. Up until this time, the baby's head represented nearly a third of his total length. Now his body will take on more human proportions.

By now, your baby's arms, legs, hands, feet, fingers, and toes are fully formed. The fingers and toes have tiny nails that reach nearly to their tips.

Bone tissue is forming rapidly, giving your baby's body increasing strength as each day passes. Your baby will become more and more active this month; his days will be filled with a great deal of tumbling, kicking, and pushing. He will frequently open and close his mouth and may even begin to suck his thumb.

During this period of growth, your baby also sleeps, perhaps up to 22 hours a day. Rest and quietness alternate with periods of vigorous activity. When he is awake, he moves and thrashes, but when he sleeps, you may not feel movement for several hours.

Even though the baby's organs are growing and maturing, it will still be several weeks before he can survive on his own outside your body. In the meantime, the placenta has been doing much of the work that your baby's organs are not yet capable of doing.

As discussed earlier, it is within the placenta that the building blocks for your baby's growth pass from your blood to your baby's blood and that his waste products pass into your body for excretion.

The placenta acts much like a screen that allows certain substances to pass through easily while keeping other substances out. For instance, the placenta allows oxygen to pass from your blood to your baby's blood and allows carbon dioxide from your baby's blood to enter your system to be removed.

The placenta can also keep some substances in your blood from entering your baby's body. Unfortunately, some substances that are potentially harmful to your baby—such as alcohol—do pass through the placenta into your baby's blood. Likewise, harmful habits like smoking and cocaine use can damage the placenta itself, making it much more difficult for your baby to obtain the oxygen and nutrients he needs. So while the placenta is capable of doing remarkable work, you need to provide both you and your baby with proper nutrition, and you need to avoid alcohol, cigarettes, and other drugs throughout your pregnancy.

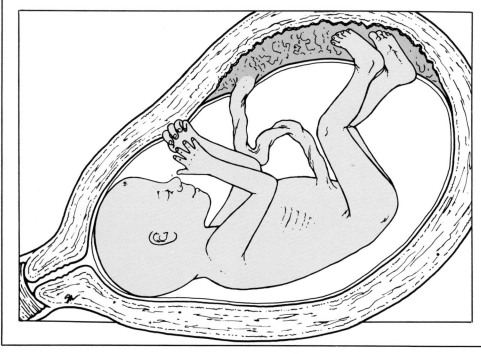

# Your Changing Body

By now, you probably know that the fluttering that you are feeling in your abdomen is not caused by indigestion or gas but rather by the movements of your baby. During the weeks ahead, these movements will become more pronounced and may even be visible as ripples and bulges that appear on your abdomen.

You may also begin to notice muscle cramps in your legs, especially toward the end of the day. This is a very common problem that begins in the middle of pregnancy and is the result of two very normal changes in your body. First, your posture has changed dramatically and your back is tipped slightly backward to compensate for the weight of your enlarging uterus. This puts a strain on the muscles in your calves and thighs and leads to leg cramps. Second, muscle cramps may result from an imbalance in the levels of calcium and phosphorus in your body. Since the baby is constantly taking calcium from your body to build his growing bones, you may become deficient in calcium. Calcium deficiency commonly leads to muscle cramps.

During the fifth month of pregnancy, many women find that their gums bleed easily after they brush their teeth. During pregnancy, the volume of blood in your body increases significantly. This increase is needed to supply the baby with vital nutrients and oxygen. As a result of this increase in your blood volume, blood vessels throughout your body, including those in your mouth and gums, become engorged. The enlarged blood vessels in your gums are easily broken with brushing.

Many women also begin to experience sinus congestion during the middle of pregnancy and may become concerned that they have an infection or an allergy. This sensation is also caused by the enlargement of blood vessels, this time within your nose and sinuses. If you do develop a runny nose or fever with your nasal congestion, however, consult your doctor.

Two other changes that you may experience during the second

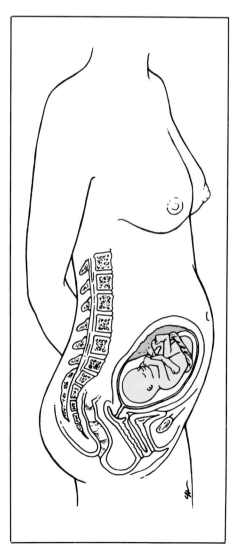

trimester are a marked increase in salivation and an altered sense of taste when eating certain foods. The reasons for these changes are not known, but they could be

## Now, you can feel your baby move.

caused by enlarged blood vessels in the tongue and mouth.

By the second trimester, most women have accepted the reality that they are going to have a baby and are looking forward to delivery day. The thrill of feeling the baby move in the uterus and of hearing the baby's heartbeat help to make his existence very real to you. You will now begin to recognize the baby as a separate person and you may find yourself wondering about your baby's personality, sex, and appearance. At this time, you may also find that you need more reassurance and affection from your husband, and you may become concerned about his safety.

The father may also be feeling a great deal of emotion at this time. He, too, may be asking himself "Will I be a good parent?" or "Will I be able to support my new family?" He may also feel that he is being left out of your life and may even unconsciously resent the baby. These feelings, too, will pass.

As a couple, you are sharing many new emotions and may be developing new needs. But because you both are unique, your reactions may differ from those of other couples and even from those of one another. It is important for both of you to be aware of these new emotions and needs and to offer each other love and support.

# How Will I Know if Something is Wrong?

## If you ever experience any of these "warning signs," notify your doctor immediately.

It is the hope and dream of all parents to experience a normal pregnancy and bring home a healthy baby. Although the majority of pregnancies *are* uneventful, some involve complications that may range from minor to life-threatening—for the mother, the baby, or both.

Complications of pregnancy may develop gradually or suddenly and without warning. One objective of prenatal care, therefore, is to promptly diagnose and treat these complications.

In this section, we will describe the "warning signs" of pregnancy—signs that may indicate that a complication is developing. If you ever experience any of these warning signs, notify your doctor immediately.

**Any Vaginal Bleeding or Spotting.** Normally, after your last menstrual period you should have no more vaginal bleeding until the delivery of your baby. If you do experience bleeding or spotting at any time during your pregnancy, contact your doctor or hospital immediately.

Bleeding that occurs during the first trimester may indicate that a miscarriage is occurring or that the pregnancy may be located outside the uterus—for example, in the fallopian tube (called an ectopic pregnancy).

Bleeding or spotting that occurs in the second or third trimester may indicate a problem with the placenta. In some cases, the placenta may begin to separate from the wall of the uterus and cause bleeding. This condition is called placental abruption. In other cases, the placenta—which should normally be located high up in the uterus—may grow down too low and cover the opening of the cervix (called placenta previa). Bleeding may then occur from exposed blood vessels over the canal of the cervix. These problems are usually diagnosed with the aid of ultrasound.

**Severe Cramping or Sharp Abdominal Pain.** This is another sign that may indicate that the placenta has begun to separate from the wall of the uterus. If you experience such cramping or pain, call your doctor immediately.

**Pain or Burning During Urination.** Bacterial infection of the bladder and kidneys is more common during pregnancy. Severe infection is not only painful, but it may also cause you to go into labor prematurely. Therefore, it is extremely important to call your doctor if you experience either pain or a burning sensation when you urinate. Do not attempt to treat yourself with home remedies.

**Fever or Chills.** If you develop a fever of over 100 degrees or experience chills, this may be a sign of infection. Even though most fevers are caused by a "cold" or the flu, your doctor will need to explore the possibility of pneumonia or kidney infection. If your amniotic sac has broken, fever and chills may indicate an infection of the amniotic fluid—a serious condition that will require antibiotics and delivery of the baby.

**Rupture of the Amniotic Sac or Leakage of Fluid.** When the amniotic sac breaks, some women have a sudden gush of fluid from the vagina while others may have only a slight leak. In the majority of pregnancies, labor begins within 24 hours of the rupture of the amniotic sac. Sometimes, however, the amniotic sac may rupture prematurely.

When the amniotic sac breaks, the protective seal around the baby is broken and bacteria from your vagina may enter the amniotic fluid. This can cause a serious infection in the baby and placenta within a few hours. Therefore, you should call your doctor immediately—whether or not you are near your estimated delivery

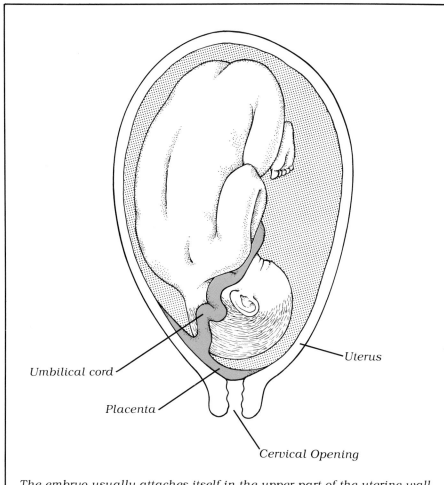

*The embryo usually attaches itself in the upper part of the uterine wall, but sometimes implantation takes place in a lower location. As the placenta grows, it can partially or completely cover the opening of the uterus, causing abnormal bleeding in the second or third trimester.*

Labels on image: Umbilical cord, Placenta, Uterus, Cervical Opening

the calves of the legs, become much more common. This is a serious condition, since these clots can break away and travel through the mother's bloodstream to the lungs, heart, or brain. Even if you think it is only a simple muscle strain, report any unusual leg soreness, as well as any redness, to your doctor immediately.

## This Month's Visit

During this month's office visit, your doctor will probably:

- Check your weight. By now, you will have gained about ten to 12 pounds; if you have not gained this amount, your doctor will probably advise you to increase the number of calories you consume each day.
- Check your blood pressure. Your blood pressure may be slightly lower than it was before pregnancy.
- Check your urine for sugar and protein. You should normally have neither in your urine.
- Ask about symptoms of pregnancy. You may now be experiencing leg cramps, bleeding gums, sinus congestion, and changes in your sense of taste.
- Ask you how you are feeling.
- Ask about the baby's movements. By now, you should feel the baby moving and kicking.
- Check the growth of your uterus by feeling your lower abdomen and measuring the distance from your pubic bone to the top of the uterus with a tape measure. By now, the top of your uterus should be at about the level of your navel.
- Listen for the baby's heartbeat with a doppler instrument or with a stethoscope. The baby's heart will beat about 140 to 160 times a minute.
- Perform a blood test to check your blood sugar level.

date—if you ever suspect that the sac has broken or is leaking.

**Swelling or Puffiness of the Face, Hands, and Feet.** This may be a sign that you are developing a condition called preeclampsia, also called toxemia. This complication of pregnancy is associated with abnormally high blood pressure, protein in the urine, and swelling (edema) of the face, hands, and feet. If toxemia is left untreated and becomes severe, seizures, stroke, and even death can occur.

Other warning signs that may indicate preeclampsia include:

- Continuous or severe headache
- Unexplained dizziness
- Blurred vision
- Continuous, severe, or recurrent vomiting
- Decrease in the amount of your urine

**Decreased Movement of the Baby.** In cases where an abnormality of the placenta may be developing, the baby's movements may slow down considerably or even stop. If you ever suspect that your baby is moving less than usual during the third trimester, call your doctor immediately.

**Soreness or Redness in One or Both Legs.** Because of certain changes in the blood during pregnancy, blood clots, especially in

# Catching Your Second Wind

Many women feel that the second trimester is the most pleasant period in pregnancy, since many of the discomforts of early pregnancy have passed by this time.

By the beginning of the second trimester, most of the symptoms and discomforts of early pregnancy will have passed and you'll probably be experiencing a renewed sense of energy. On the other hand, you'll also begin to develop new symptoms that are related not only to your increasing hormone levels but also to your rapidly growing baby.

## COMMON DISCOMFORTS OF THE SECOND TRIMESTER

**Backache.** This nearly universal discomfort of pregnancy occurs when your posture changes to accommodate the increased size and weight of your uterus and baby. Stress is placed on the muscles and ligaments in the lower part of the back, causing an aching sensation in this area.

Of course, there's nothing you can do about the increasing size and weight of your uterus. But the less additional stress you place on your back, the better you will feel. You may find the following suggestions useful for minimizing or relieving backache.

• Support the weight of the uterus and baby when walking, stand-

ing, and sitting by using good posture. The straighter your body, the less strain is put on your back muscles (see *For You and Your Baby*, page 84, for directions on how to maintain good posture).
• Wear comfortable shoes with a slight heel (one to one-and-a-half inches high) and good support. Avoid wearing high-heeled shoes, since they will cause you to arch your back and strain your muscles.
• Whenever you must reach down for anything, bend your knees and squat down, keeping your back straight. Do not bend your back. Pull whatever you are reaching for close to your chest. Then use your leg muscles to push yourself up to a standing position.
• Avoid standing for extended periods of time. Sit down when you can and assume a good sitting posture (see page 85).
• When you are rising from bed or from a chair, use the muscles of your arms and legs to push yourself up rather than using your back muscles to pull yourself up.
• Avoid heavy lifting or pushing that may strain your back.

• Sleep on a firm mattress. Placing a board under the mattress may also help.
• A heating pad and a gentle massage can help relieve back pain.
• Don't take any medication without your doctor's approval.
• A good exercise program to strengthen your back and abdominal muscles may help to prevent backache; discuss specific exercises with your doctor or childbirth educator.

Back pain, especially if it is constant and severe, may be a symptom of a more serious problem such as a kidney infection or a slipped disc. If your back pain is not relieved by these simple measures, call your doctor.

**Skin Changes.** Pregnant women commonly develop a variety of skin changes, including itching and dryness, increased perspiration and oiliness, and increased pigmentation on the face and abdomen.

Dryness and itching are best relieved by applying moisturizing creams or lotions regularly, especially after bathing. Some women feel that cocoa-butter products are best.

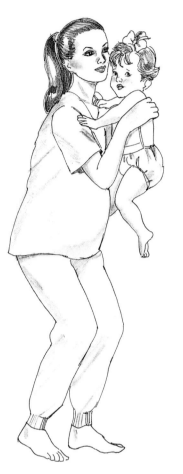

*When lifting a child (or object) from the floor, bend your knees and keep your back straight. Hold the child close to your chest and use your leg muscles to push yourself up to a standing position.*

Increased oiliness of the skin sometimes causes a mild outbreak of acne. If this occurs, cleanse your skin frequently with a mild soap.

Some women experience increased perspiration throughout pregnancy. Aside from cleansing frequently and using deodorant/antiperspirant, there is little that can be done to relieve this problem.

Increased pigmentation of the skin is common and occurs when hormones stimulate certain cells in the lower layers of the skin. Although nothing can be done to stop this from occurring during pregnancy, applying cosmetics and avoiding direct exposure to sunlight will help lighten the areas of darkened skin. After pregnancy, these skin changes disappear.

**Stretch Marks.** Beginning in the second trimester, you may develop stretch marks on the skin of your abdomen, breasts, and thighs. There is no way to prevent stretch marks from occurring, but the use of lanolin skin lotions may help. These red marks will never completely disappear after pregnancy, but they will fade to thin silvery lines that are much less noticeable.

**Bleeding Gums.** You may find that your gums bleed easily when you brush your teeth or floss. Since your gums are receiving an increased supply of blood and are now slightly swollen, they can be injured quite easily. This is a harmless problem that cannot be completely avoided. Using a soft-bristled toothbrush and avoiding harsh scrubbing may help.

**Appetite Changes.** Many women report a change in their sense of taste when eating certain foods during pregnancy. The exact reason for this is not known; it may be related to the increased blood supply to the tongue, which may affect the taste buds.

Many women also report an aversion to certain foods and food smells during pregnancy. Even though they may have once enjoyed them, the smell or even the sight of certain foods may lead to nausea and sometimes even vomiting. The cause of this is not known. It is best relieved by avoiding such foods and smells whenever possible.

Increased salivation is also common during pregnancy and is probably related to the expanded size of blood vessels in the mouth. It is a harmless problem that may also alter the taste of certain foods.

**Headache.** During pregnancy, most headaches are caused by relatively harmless problems such as tension, sinus congestion, or a cold. Simple measures, such as massaging the neck and shoulder muscles or lying down in a quiet room and applying ice packs to your forehead, will cure most simple headaches. Avoid taking medications without first trying these simple techniques; consult your doctor before taking any medication. Mild, occasional headaches are of little concern.

If headaches are severe or continuous, they may signal a more serious problem and should be reported to your doctor immediately. For example, severe or continuous headache may be caused by a sinus infection or an abscessed tooth. During the third trimester, severe headache may be a symptom of preeclampsia.

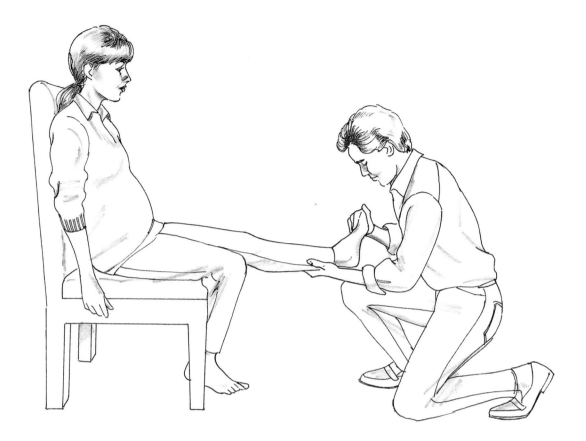

*To relieve a leg cramp, sit down and extend your leg with your toes pointed upward. Then have your partner gently push your toes toward you to stretch your calf muscle.*

If you have a history of migraine headaches, your migraines may become more severe during pregnancy. On the other hand, some women report that their migraines become less severe and less frequent.

**Leg Cramps.** Painful cramps in the muscles of the legs may result from either an imbalance of calcium and phosphorus in your body or from the strain placed on the leg muscles by poor posture.

Milk is a major source of calcium; it is important that you not omit it from your diet during pregnancy. Carbonated beverages, on the other hand, contain phosphorus, and drinking too many of these may lead to an overabundance of phosphorus in your body.

If you do develop painful leg cramps, try increasing your milk and milk-product intake and eliminating carbonated beverages, replacing them with juices, tea, or water. If these measures fail, discuss the problem with your doctor, since she can prescribe calcium supplements or safe medications that reduce your phosphorus levels.

Muscle cramps may also be due to the strain caused by poor posture. Pay close attention to the alignment of your body when you are standing (see page 84). If a painful cramp does occur, sit down and pull up on your toes (or extend your leg and have someone gently push your toes toward you) to flex your foot and stretch your calf

muscles. This will often relieve the cramp on the spot.

**Heartburn.** There are three reasons why you may develop heartburn. First, the hormone progesterone, which is produced by the placenta, slows the action of your digestive system and causes the stomach to empty into the intestines more slowly. Second, progesterone relaxes the tight band of muscle between the esophagus and stomach. And finally, the enlarging uterus pushes up on the stomach and decreases its capacity to hold food. All of these factors combine to allow food and stomach acid to back up into your esophagus and produce a burning sensation. The following measures may help you relieve or prevent heartburn.

- Eat several small meals instead of three large ones during the day.
- Avoid lying down within the two hours following eating or drinking.
- Sleep with your head and back elevated on several pillows.
- Avoid spicy foods.

If these methods fail to relieve heartburn, call your doctor and she can recommend a safe antacid that will coat the stomach and esophagus and reduce irritation and pain. Never use baking soda as a home remedy, since it has a very high salt content.

**Indigestion and Gas.** These are also very common discomforts of pregnancy and are related to the slowing down of your digestive system caused by progesterone. The same methods used to relieve heartburn may also be tried for indigestion and gas. Eating several smaller meals instead of three large meals each day and chewing your food thoroughly may help prevent gas formation in the stomach and intestines. You should also try to avoid gas-producing foods such as beans, onions, and cabbage.

Indigestion may also sometimes be a symptom of a more serious condition, such as gallstones, so if simple home treatments do not relieve your digestive discomfort, call your doctor.

## PSYCHOLOGICAL CHANGES

During the second trimester, you will probably develop a sense of general well-being. The fear of miscarriage has usually disappeared, and the physical discomforts of the first trimester have diminished. Most women feel that the second trimester is the most pleasant period in pregnancy.

The most overwhelming event during the second trimester occurs at the time of fetal movement. With this nearly constant reminder of the baby growing within your uterus, you may begin to feel an increased dependency toward your partner. You may have more needs than usual, and you may worry about whether your partner will be available, interested, and able to support you during this time of change.

During pregnancy, you may find that you are much more vulnerable to certain fears and concerns. For example, pregnant women are often more anxious about the possibility of bodily harm. Things ordinarily taken for

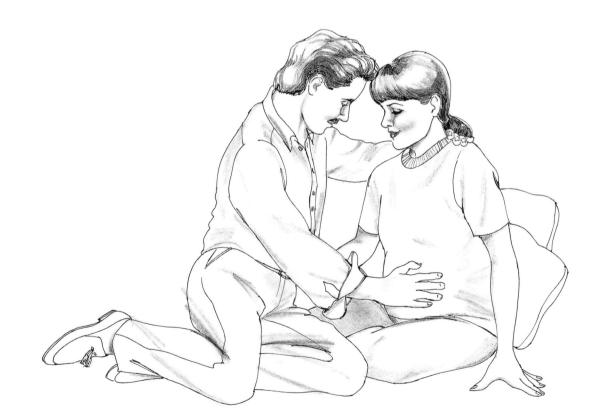

granted, such as riding in a car or engaging in physical activity, may provoke some anxiety.

These anxieties will often surface in your dreams. Dreams may be realistic representations of your fears, or they may take the form of nightmares. Dreaming about your worries is normal and may help you to deal with your concerns during the day. Be reassured that dreams usually do not represent life as it really is—or as it will be once the baby is born.

There is a progression of changing themes in dreams that may occur throughout your pregnancy. Dreams about pregnancy and babies often begin in the first trimester. Uncertainties about your new role as a mother may surface in dreams about not being able to care properly for your baby. Such dreams are normal.

Pregnant women often dream about being trapped, and in many ways this is a direct representation of fears and concerns about the future. Especially if you have worked outside the home, you may be frightened about what having a baby will do to your ability to maintain outside interests.

Many mothers dream about having a child of one sex or the other. These dreams may reflect your preference for a child of a particular sex, as well as your concerns about your own sexual identity.

Another common theme in dreams is looking for a child or losing a child. Dreams about such loss usually occur toward the end of pregnancy, when you begin to anticipate the delivery of your own child. In reality, a loss is about to occur—the loss of the fetus within you when he becomes your baby at delivery.

Assault is another theme that may occur in your dreams about pregnancy; it reflects your worry that if you were to be assaulted or injured, the consequences might be harmful to your baby as well as to yourself. Also, as the pregnancy continues and your body enlarges, you may worry that you will not be able to react quickly in a dangerous situation.

Perhaps the most relevant anxiety about assault that a pregnant woman has to deal with is the loss of control over her body. Clearly, you are not in control of

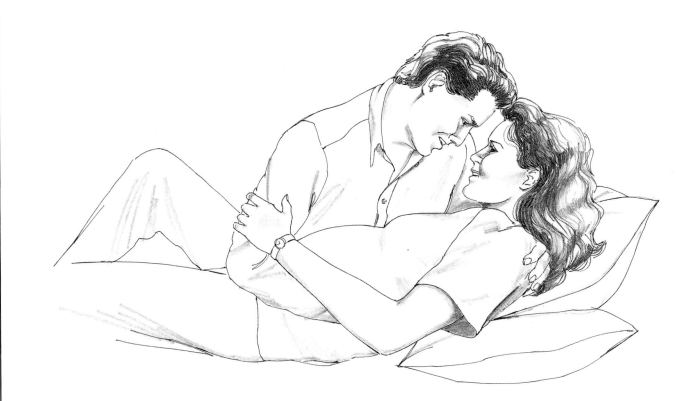

your body's changes during pregnancy. Especially for the first-time mother, these assault dreams may reflect your fears about what labor and delivery will be like. Then, too, the assault dreams may reflect your feelings about the "stranger" who is within your body.

Remember, having these frightening dreams is normal and should not worry you. In fact, it is because of the love you feel for the baby inside you that you are concerned about his fragility; that concern, which is reflected in your dreams, is not unusual at all.

## SEXUAL RELATIONS

During the second trimester, both vaginal lubrication and blood flow to the pelvic area increase. These changes, plus the easing of the nausea and breast sensitivity that developed in the first trimester, may increase your desire for sexual relations.

You may wonder, however, if your husband still considers you attractive. Some women and men, particularly in this weight-conscious society, associate weight gain with unattractiveness. Talking to each other about this should help alleviate many of your fears and misconceptions so that you and your partner can enjoy a healthy sexual relationship during your second trimester.

## YOUR DEVELOPING BABY'S HEALTH

Safety issues continue to be of major importance for the pregnant woman during the second trimester. Even though your baby's organs have formed and he is becoming more resistant to harm, you must still be concerned about physical injury, certain infections, and exposure to hazardous substances.

**Seat Belts.** You should always wear a seat belt with a shoulder restraint when you are driving or riding in a car. The lap belt should

be placed snugly across your hips *below* your abdomen. The shoulder restraint should be placed *above* the abdomen and between your breasts. Never place a seat belt directly over your abdomen during pregnancy.

**Hair Coloring and Permanents.** At this time, there is no evidence to indicate that the chemicals used for hair coloring and permanents are dangerous to your baby. On the other hand, they have not been proven entirely safe

---

> When using
> household cleaners
> and polishes,
> always wear
> rubber gloves.

---

either. Since all of these chemicals can be absorbed by the body through the skin, some may find their way to the developing baby. Furthermore, most women find that permanents performed during pregnancy do not "take" well anyway and often fall out within a week.

**Cosmetics.** Like the chemicals used on hair, little is known about the safety of cosmetics. Those that contain small amounts of mercury are known to be hazardous to some women, and there is certainly reason to believe that they might harm the baby as well. Ask your obstetrician or dermatologist about safe cosmetics, and use them sparingly.

**Aerosol Sprays.** Hair sprays, underarm deodorants, furniture polish, and disinfectants often come in aerosol cans that also contain substances called fluorocarbons. These substances are generally thought to be harmless to people, but their effects on a developing baby are not known. Try substituting pump containers for aerosols during pregnancy.

**Paints and Paint Fumes.** Certain potentially harmful substances used in paints can be absorbed through the skin and inhaled from fumes. Avoid using paints and paint thinners while you are pregnant and avoid rooms that have been freshly painted until they have aired out well.

**Insect and Weed Killers.** Avoid any contact with these substances, since they can be absorbed by the skin and enter the baby's bloodstream.

**Cleaners and Polishes.** Chemicals contained in household cleaners and polishes are also readily absorbed through the skin and could potentially enter your developing baby's bloodstream. When using these substances, always wear gloves and avoid breathing the fumes.

**Infections.** During the second trimester, infections in the mother continue to pose a serious threat to the baby. Be certain to report to your doctor immediately any rash, high fever, unusual vaginal discharge, skin ulcers, or cold or flu symptoms that do not go away with simple home remedies.

**Drugs.** Even though your baby's organs have formed and he is growing rapidly, there are still many drugs that pose a hazard to his well-being and development. Make certain that you never use a drug during pregnancy, even those that may be purchased without a prescription, unless approved by your doctor. The following are drugs that may affect your baby throughout pregnancy.

*Aspirin and Aspirin Substitutes.* When aspirin is taken by a woman shortly before delivery, it can cause blood-clotting abnormalities in her newborn baby. During a routine delivery, the baby's head and other organs are subject to a great deal of pressure. If the baby's blood clots normally, this pressure will not lead to injury. If, however, his blood clots more slowly because of the effects of aspirin, he may develop large bruises under his skin, or worse, bleeding beneath his skull bones or within his internal organs.

Since dangerous bleeding may occur in the newborn, and since aspirin has not been proven absolutely safe at other times during pregnancy, avoid all aspirin and aspirin-containing drugs

> ## Do not take any drugs, even those that are available without a prescription, before checking with your doctor.

during your pregnancy unless your doctor directs you otherwise.

Nonaspirin pain relievers and anti-inflammatory agents, such as acetaminophen and ibuprofen, have also not been proven absolutely safe during pregnancy. Therefore, it is wise to avoid these "aspirin substitutes" throughout pregnancy unless your doctor directs you otherwise.

Many common drugs that you can purchase without a prescription for headaches, colds, and sinus congestion contain aspirin or an aspirin substitute. Be sure to read the label on any medication before you use it to be sure it does not contain one of these substances.

*Sleeping Pills.* Pills that you can purchase without a prescription to help you sleep have not been proven absolutely safe for use during pregnancy. Since sleeping pills are rarely necessary to maintain your health, avoid their use during pregnancy. Try a warm bath, a warm drink, a gentle massage, or other simple techniques if you are having trouble falling asleep.

*Water Pills (diuretics).* Drugs that increase urine production are commonly used by women to relieve swelling that may occur before the menstrual period. The use of these drugs during pregnancy has been associated with abnormalities of certain internal organs in the newborn. Unless advised by your doctor, never use water pills during pregnancy.

*Antibiotics.* Some antibiotics, such as penicillin and ampicillin, are safe for use during pregnancy. Certain other common antibiotics, however, may seriously affect the baby. For example, the use of tetracycline during pregnancy has been associated with abnormalities of bone growth in the baby and may also lead to a permanent brown staining of the baby's teeth.

The use of sulfa drugs, another medication commonly used to treat infection, may cause the baby to have severe jaundice (yellow skin) and other abnormalities at birth.

**Hot Tubs and Saunas.** A high body temperature in the mother has also been found to be dangerous to the developing baby. If you are outside on a hot day, even if the temperature is over 100 degrees, your body will perspire and your temperature will usually not rise above normal as long as you drink plenty of fluids and avoid strenuous activity or exposure to direct sunlight for long periods of time.

If you are in a hot tub or a sauna, however, your body's cooling mechanism may not be able to keep your temperature in the normal range; your body temperature may easily reach 105 degrees, which is potentially harmful to your baby. If you are pregnant, avoid using hot tubs and saunas, as well as any other activity that may significantly raise your body temperature.

## FOR YOUR COMFORT

**Clothing.** During the first three months of your pregnancy, you were probably able to wear your usual clothing, since the size of your uterus had not yet affected your shape or waistline. After the third month of pregnancy, however, you will need to wear clothing that will fit your new contours.

Fortunately, maternity clothing today is available in a wide variety of attractive styles for both business

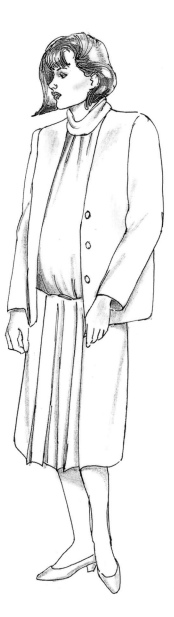

and leisure. Whether you purchase, borrow, or make your maternity clothing, chances are you'll find patterns and styles that will suit your tastes and your needs for work and leisure. What's more, many maternity dresses, slacks, and tops are designed for use even after the baby is born, which will increase the usefulness of your new wardrobe. To help keep costs down, try borrowing some pieces from friends who have been pregnant or try invading your husband's closet for loose-fitting shirts and jackets.

When choosing maternity clothing, you will usually wear the same dress size and top size as you did before pregnancy. In the design of the clothing, the manufacturer will have taken into consideration the size of your abdomen, so if you wore a size eight before pregnancy, you will still be able to wear a size eight maternity dress.

When fitting slacks, however, you may need slacks that are one to two sizes larger than the size you wore before pregnancy (although many maternity slacks come with an expandable waistline, you may find a larger size will fit you more comfortably around the thighs). For example, if you wore size eight slacks before pregnancy, you will probably need a size ten or size 12 during pregnancy.

You will also find that wearing clothing that is tight around your abdomen will be uncomfortable and will interfere with your breathing. Many current styles of maternity skirts and slacks, therefore, have an adjustable waistline or expandable front panel that helps to relieve pressure on your abdomen. You may also want to choose more outfits that are suspended from the shoulders, such as jumpers, overalls, and dresses.

Your new clothing should not only be comfortable, but it should help you feel good about your new appearance. A well-chosen wardrobe will do wonders for your self-image during pregnancy.

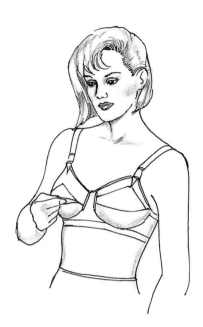

*Some maternity bras have flaps on the cups, making them suitable for breast-feeding once the baby is born.*

**Brassieres.** Throughout pregnancy, you will need a well-fitting bra to support your enlarging breasts. This will not only increase your comfort, but it may also reduce the development of stretch marks. Choose a maternity bra of the uplift or sling type that lifts the breasts upward and inward. Avoid any type that flattens the breasts.

Toward the end of pregnancy, you may wish to purchase a bra with flaps over the front that may be used for breast-feeding after the baby is born.

**Maternity Girdle.** A girdle is generally unnecessary during pregnancy and may in some cases restrict your breathing. However, some women, especially those who have had children before, find that a girdle provides additional comfort by helping to support the back and abdomen.

If you do wish to wear a girdle, make certain that you purchase

one that is specifically designed for pregnant women. In addition, make sure the girdle fits well and is not too tight around the legs or abdomen.

**Stockings and Panty Hose.** During pregnancy, it is important that you not restrict the flow of blood in your legs, since this can lead to swelling, varicose veins, and

---

## Avoid wearing clothing that wraps tightly around your legs or abdomen.

---

even worse, the formation of blood clots. Never wear stockings, garters, or panty girdles that wrap tightly around your legs. In general, well-fitting maternity panty hose are your best choice.

**Shoes.** Your choice of shoes during pregnancy will affect both your comfort and your safety. Since your posture will undergo changes, it will be important for you to avoid shoes that will put excessive strain on your lower back and leg muscles.

High-heeled shoes cause an exaggeration of the swayback caused by the protruding abdomen. They also increase your risk of twisting an ankle, slipping, or falling.

A reasonable heel height of one to one-and-one-half inches is suggested (this heel height is even preferable to flats). The shoe should also provide good support and have a closed heel instead of a sling back. Avoid thongs and sandals, which may cause you to twist your ankle or fall. When purchasing new shoes, you may want to buy a slightly larger pair in anticipation of the swelling in the feet that commonly occurs during pregnancy, especially toward the end of the day or after you've been sitting for an extended period of time.

# Your Growing Baby

During his sixth month, your baby is continuing to add weight and length, and his tiny, thin body is beginning to fill out. The baby is now between 11 and 14 inches long and weighs one-and-a-quarter to one-and-a-half pounds. Quite a growth spurt in only one month!

By now, your baby's features have undergone considerable refinement. His face is well defined and resembles that of a newborn. Eyelashes and eyebrows are quite distinct, although the eyelids remain closed.

Other small details are also being formed this month. Fingers and toes continue to develop a newborn appearance. Fingerprints and footprints—which are unique to each individual and which will remain throughout life—are just beginning to form. Lanugo hair still covers your baby's body, but dark, coarse hair is already making its appearance on the scalp.

Even though he is rapidly filling out his body, your baby's skin during his sixth month is still red and wrinkled, with very little fat

---

### Your baby may now respond to loud noise.

---

beneath it. Over the next three months, more and more fat will form under the skin to eventually give baby a slightly chubby appearance.

During this month, a baby's skin develops a protective covering called vernix caseosa. This whitish-yellow, cheesy substance sticks to his skin with the help of the lanugo and forms a thick barrier that protects the skin from the amniotic fluid. By the ninth month, almost all of this coating will disappear, although some babies may still have some around the creases of their arms and legs when they are born.

During his sixth month, scientists believe that your baby is probably becoming aware of his environment. His tiny brain is beginning to function and his ears and eyes have developed to the point where they can sense things inside and outside your body. For example, you may become aware that your baby moves and kicks after a loud noise, such as the crash of a pan or dish hitting the floor. In some cases, you may also find that the baby stops moving in response to quiet, soothing music. It is also believed that he may actually be able to see some faint light as it passes through the walls of your abdomen and uterus.

Your baby is now floating in nearly a quart of amniotic fluid. He is connected to the placenta by the umbilical cord like an astronaut in space connected to the mother ship.

The clear, watery amniotic fluid serves many purposes for your developing baby. It helps to keep his body temperature normal, it provides an environment in which he can move about freely and exercise his growing muscles, and it helps to cushion him from any injury that may occur to your abdomen.

Just prior to delivery, the amniotic sac will break, releasing its fluid into your vagina. In some cases, it will break on its own; in others, your doctor may purposely break it with a special instrument.

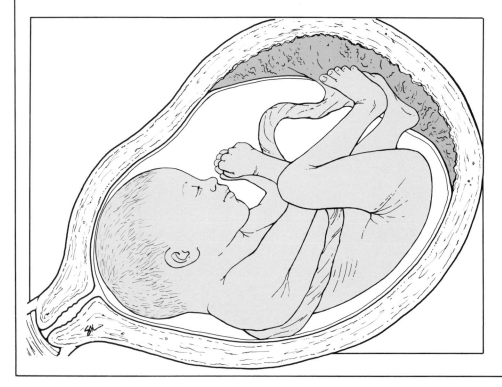

# MONTH

# Your Changing Body

Several changes will occur in your body during the sixth month of pregnancy, and, as before, they will be caused by your increasing hormone levels and your enlarging uterus.

By now, you will probably have experienced heartburn. This is a normal discomfort of pregnancy and occurs for several reasons. First, the hormone progesterone slows the action of the entire digestive system, including the stomach. Since it now takes a longer time for the stomach to empty its contents into the intestines below, there is more chance of an upward flow—or regurgitation—of food back up into your esophagus (the tube through which food travels from your mouth to your stomach). This food, which is mixed with stomach acids, is highly irritating to the esophagus. It is this irritation that causes you to have the burning sensation in the middle of your chest.

The second reason you may experience heartburn has to do with the tight band of muscle, called a sphincter, at the point where the esophagus connects to the stomach. Normally, this band of muscle tightens after you eat and prevents food from re-entering your esophagus. The increase in the level of progesterone that occurs during pregnancy, however, can cause this sphincter to weaken, allowing further regurgitation of food.

Finally, as your uterus enlarges, it pushes up firmly against the stomach and may actually force food up into the esophagus.

You may also be noticing several additional changes in your skin. The first of these are stretch marks, which may begin to develop on your abdomen, breasts, and thighs. These slightly indented, silvery-red streaks are the result of ruptured fibers in the skin caused by the enlarging uterus, the increase in breast tissue, and the increased accumulation of fat in the thighs.

Not all pregnant women develop stretch marks. The tendency to develop stretch marks

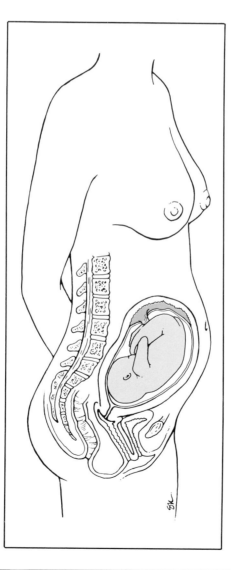

seems to run in the mother's side of the family. To get an idea of whether you will develop stretch marks and to what extent, look at your mother or sisters. If they didn't develop stretch marks during pregnancy, then there is a good chance that you won't either, and vice versa. Any stretch marks that do develop will gradually fade into thin, silvery lines within a few months after delivery.

Another common skin change of pregnancy is hyperpigmentation. Estrogen produced by the placenta indirectly stimulates skin cells to produce increasing amounts of dark pigment. This pigment then causes darkening of the skin in certain parts of your body. The areola, the dark skin that surrounds the breast nipple, usually becomes darker. Blotchy, brown patches—called chloasma or "mask of pregnancy"—often develop on the face. You may also notice a dark line, called linea nigra, running down the middle of your abdomen from your navel to your vagina. These pigment changes almost always fade away after delivery.

During the sixth month of pregnancy, you will also probably begin to notice occasional contractions of your uterus. These so-called Braxton Hicks contractions (named after Dr. Braxton Hicks, an English physician who first described them) are transient, irregular, and nonpainful contractions of the uterus (unlike the stronger, more frequent, and painful contractions that signal labor). You may first notice these as a tight feeling in your lower abdomen. Braxton Hicks contractions will occur throughout the remainder of pregnancy and will generally become more frequent.

# Should I Worry About Rh Incompatibility?

## Once a leading cause of death in babies throughout the world, Rh incompatibility can now be prevented through routine prenatal blood testing and the use of certain drugs.

Another area in which rapid advances in obstetrics have led to more healthy newborn babies is Rh incompatibility. Once a disease that was a leading cause of death in babies throughout the world, Rh incompatibility can now be easily prevented through routine prenatal blood testing and the use of certain drugs.

### What is the Rh Factor?

Approximately 87 percent of white persons and 93 percent of black persons are born with a substance on their blood cells known as the Rh factor, so called because a similar substance is found on the blood cells of rhesus monkeys. Individuals who have this factor on their blood cells are called Rh positive; those without it are called

| During First Pregnancy | At Delivery | After Delivery | During Subsequent Pregnancy |

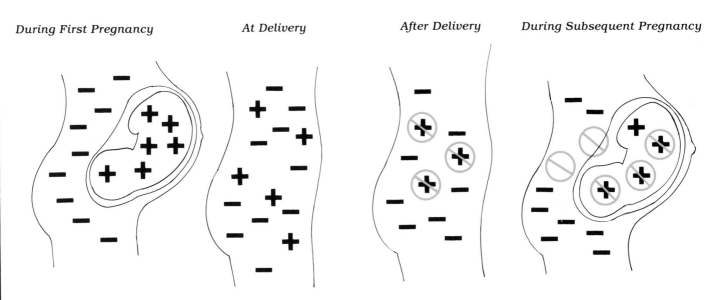

*During First Pregnancy:* The Rh− mother carries her first Rh+ baby. No problems generally occur in this first baby. *At Delivery:* Some of the baby's Rh+ blood enters the mother's bloodstream. *After Delivery:* If the mother does not receive a special serum, her body makes antibodies that destroy Rh+ blood cells. These antibodies remain in the mother's bloodstream. *During Subsequent Pregnancy:* The mother's antibodies attack the blood cells of any subsequent Rh+ babies.

Rh negative. The presence of the Rh factor is inherited from one's parents.

**When Does the Rh Factor Cause Problems?** The genes that a baby receives from his parents at conception dictate whether or not he will be Rh positive or Rh negative. Normally, during labor and delivery, some of the baby's blood will escape from the placenta and enter the mother's blood. If both the mother and the fetus are Rh positive or if both are Rh negative, this leakage of fetal blood will cause no problems.

If the mother's blood is Rh negative and the baby's blood is Rh positive (the baby would have received the gene for the Rh factor from his father), however, a problem can occur. When the baby's Rh-positive blood enters the mother's Rh-negative blood during delivery, the mother's blood considers the baby's Rh factor to be a foreign substance. The mother's body then begins to form antibodies to get rid of this foreign substance.

Antibodies are normally formed in the body in response to foreign substances—usually bacteria and viruses that may be harmful. These antibodies act by destroying the foreign substance, thus protecting the body against their harmful effects. A person who forms antibodies against a particular substance is called "sensitized" to that substance.

When an Rh-negative mother gives birth to her first Rh-positive baby, she is likely to become sensitized to the Rh factor. That first Rh-positive baby is usually unaffected.

However, the mother's body keeps the antibodies against Rh-positive blood for life. If she becomes pregnant with an Rh-positive baby again, this fetus may be affected. During this subsequent pregnancy, the mother's antibodies may cross the placenta and begin destroying the baby's Rh-positive blood cells while the baby is still in the uterus. This can lead to anemia, heart failure, and even stillbirth.

**Can Rh Incompatibility be Prevented?** About 20 years ago, a substance was developed that could protect a mother from becoming sensitized to Rh-positive blood. This substance, called Rh0 (D) immune globulin, is injected into the Rh-negative mother shortly after she delivers an Rh-positive baby and destroys any Rh-positive blood cells that may have entered her blood. After a mother has received this injection, she will not become sensitized and will not have to worry about Rh complications developing in her next baby.

An Rh-negative woman can become sensitized to Rh-positive blood in situations other than childbirth. For example, if she has an abortion or a miscarriage and the fetus was Rh positive, fetal blood may escape into her bloodstream and she may become sensitized. Also, after removal of an ectopic pregnancy (a pregnancy that develops in an abnormal location such as the fallopian tube), she may become sensitized. A transfusion of Rh-positive blood into an Rh-negative woman (which rarely occurs today) may cause antibodies against Rh-positive blood to form.

Since it is difficult and sometimes impossible to determine the Rh factor of the fetus after a miscarriage, abortion, or removal of an ectopic pregnancy, all Rh-negative women who undergo any of these processes are automatically given an injection of the immune globulin.

During your first prenatal office visit, your doctor will perform a blood test to determine if you have Rh-negative or Rh-positive blood. If you are Rh negative, your doctor will also perform another blood test to determine if you have antibodies that will destroy Rh-positive blood; that test will probably be repeated during the third trimester of your pregnancy.

If a pregnant woman does carry antibodies against the Rh factor, an amniocentesis can be performed to determine if the fetus is being affected. In the rare instances when serious problems in the fetus are detected, the baby will be delivered immediately. If it is determined that the fetus is too young to survive outside the mother's body, a blood transfusion may be performed to replace the fetus' Rh-positive blood with Rh-negative blood.

## This Month's Visit

During this month's office visit, your doctor will probably:

- Check your weight. By now, you will have gained about 14 to 16 pounds.
- Check your blood pressure. It may be slightly below what it was before pregnancy.
- Check your urine for sugar and protein. Normally, you should have neither of these in your urine.
- Ask about symptoms of pregnancy. You may now be experiencing heartburn and occasional Braxton Hicks contractions.
- Ask you how you are feeling.
- Ask about the baby's movements. By now, the baby should be quite noticeably active throughout the day.
- Check the growth of your uterus with a tape measure. By now, the top of your uterus will be several inches above your navel.
- Listen for the baby's heartbeat with a doppler instrument or a stethoscope. The baby's heartbeat should be about 140 to 160 beats per minute.
- Offer practical advice about the third trimester and describe the sensations that you will feel when you are in labor.
- Perform no new blood tests.

# Childbirth Classes

Childbirth classes can teach you how to deal with the discomforts of labor and can give you the knowledge and confidence that help make childbirth a fulfilling experience.

The purpose of childbirth classes is to prepare future parents to deal positively with the entire experience of pregnancy, labor, and birth. Of course, every pregnancy is unique, and no one can predict exactly what will happen and how you will feel during your pregnancy and delivery. But childbirth classes can give you and your husband an idea of what to expect when you're expecting. They can help dispel myths, ease fears, and give you the knowledge and confidence that can help make childbirth a fulfilling experience for both of you.

Childbirth classes will teach you about the process of pregnancy, labor, and delivery. You will also be taught techniques to help you relax and help you deal with discomfort and pain. The more you learn about pregnancy and childbirth, the less you will fear.

Childbirth classes are available in nearly every community. Some are sponsored by hospitals or institutions, while others are taught privately by certified childbirth educators. These classes are usually inexpensive or free.

Childbirth preparation classes are usually attended during the third trimester. Most meet in the evening or on weekends, making it more convenient for you and your spouse to attend together.

Several different methods of childbirth preparation are currently popular in the United States. Each of these takes a slightly different approach to reducing the discomfort and pain of labor and delivery. Some childbirth classes teach only one method. Others provide a broader, more individualized kind of preparation, drawing from each of several different methods. The goal of these broader classes is to enable women and their partners to discover their own style for labor.

Basic to all methods of childbirth preparation is the concept that the discomfort and pain of childbirth are real, but that they can be minimized through psychological preparation. Childbirth preparation methods will not eliminate pain; rather, they teach you why pain occurs and demonstrate techniques to help you cope with it.

The following are the most commonly taught methods of childbirth preparation. At the end of this section, you will find tips for choosing the class that's right for you.

**Lamaze Method.** The Lamaze method of childbirth preparation is the most popular and widely used method in the United States today. This method is named after French physician Fernand Lamaze, who believed that by concentrating on a specific distracting stimulus during labor (such as staring at a particular spot or breathing in a controlled fashion) a pregnant woman can "block" the transmission of pain impulses from the uterus to the brain.

This method, also called "psychoprophylaxis," involves training or conditioning a woman to respond to her contractions by relaxing. Your "labor coach" (the individual you choose to help you through labor and delivery) is an important part of the Lamaze method. During the classes, he or she will be trained to help you consciously relax and help you use specific breathing patterns to take your mind off your contractions.

The Lamaze method also involves certain physical means of decreasing painful sensations, such as light massage (called effleurage) on the surface of your abdomen and back.

Since training and conditioning form the basis of the Lamaze method, it is necessary for you and your "coach" to spend time every day practicing the techniques that you learn in class. The more you practice, the more effective the method will become. Eventually, you should automatically respond

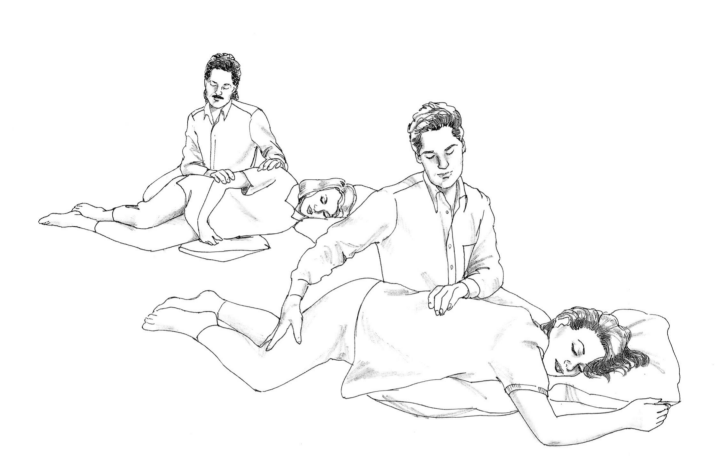

to a certain stimulus with specific breathing patterns and relaxation.

It should be emphasized that the Lamaze method is not the same as natural childbirth—that is, childbirth without pain medication. Not all women who use the Lamaze method will have the same type of delivery experience. Many women, for reasons of personal preference or medical necessity, will use some form of pain medication or anesthesia during their labor and delivery. Lamaze training is intended to help you cope with pain, not act as a substitute when pain medication is necessary. Accepting pain medication does not mean that you are a failure.

**Bradley Method.** Another common method of childbirth preparation is the Bradley method, named after obstetrician Robert Bradley. Unlike Lamaze, the Bradley method emphasizes true natural childbirth—that is, giving birth without using any drugs.

The Bradley method stresses working in harmony with the body. It prepares the woman to experience the intensity and pleasure of birth by using deep relaxation techniques and by tuning in to her body's sensations instead of using certain breathing patterns to distract her from her labor pains.

Certain fitness exercises are also part of the Bradley method. For

example, pelvic rocking exercises (see *For You and Your Baby*, page 54), are used to reduce pressure in the pelvic area and increase the flexibility of the lower back.

The Bradley method is often referred to as "husband-coached childbirth," since the father plays such a major role in maintaining the mother's deep relaxation. The father is asked to observe the mother's breathing patterns as she sleeps so that he can help her to breathe in a similar relaxed fashion during labor.

Childbirth educators who teach the Bradley method believe that true natural childbirth can take place if the parents are properly prepared. This method is especially well suited for couples who intend to give birth at home or in a free-standing birthing center.

**Dick-Read Method.** The Dick-Read method of childbirth preparation evolved from the teachings of Grantly Dick-Read, an English obstetrician. He identified what is called the fear-tension-pain cycle, emphasizing that fear causes tension, which leads to unnecessary pain. Because this pain causes further fear and tension, the cycle repeats itself.

From this observation, Dr. Dick-Read devised a method of childbirth preparation that attempts to break the fear-tension-pain cycle. This method involves teaching the mother why pain occurs in order to help relieve her fears. It also involves breathing exercises, which are designed to help the mother release tension during labor, and certain physical exercises, which help prepare her muscles and joints for the process of labor.

Today, childbirth educators who teach the Dick-Read method emphasize that the pregnant woman should work in harmony with labor; she should relax and breathe in response to her body's demands, instead of according to a set schedule.

Since the Dick-Read method prepares women for unmedicated or natural childbirth, it is also well suited for those planning a home birth or those using a birthing center.

**Kitzinger Method.** Another method of childbirth preparation is the Kitzinger method, developed by English anthropologist Sheila Kitzinger. This form of childbirth preparation is not generally taught as a separate method, but rather is incorporated into the teachings of childbirth educators who primarily teach other formal methods.

Frequently called "psychosexual preparation," this method teaches that childbirth is part of the wide spectrum of sexuality in a woman's life. Exercises are therefore described in terms of normal processes of the body, and emphasis is placed on working in harmony with these processes.

Another major part of the Kitzinger method is the use of a variety of techniques for relaxation, including gentle massage and mental imagery to develop awareness of the body.

**Leboyer Technique.** Though not a method of childbirth preparation, the Leboyer concept of "birth

---

## The more effort you put into finding a class that's right for you, the more you'll get out of it.

---

without violence" is commonly discussed in childbirth classes.

Dr. Leboyer, a French obstetrician, developed the concept of "gentle" delivery, which is designed to make birth less traumatic for the baby. He advocated a warm, quiet room with dim lights for the birth and a warm bath for the baby shortly after delivery.

In this way, he felt that the baby could be helped into a gentle and calm transition from life in the uterus to life outside the mother's body.

**Choosing a Class.** Childbirth classes are designed to make childbirth a more fulfilling experience for you and your husband, so it pays to select the class carefully. You'll want to find a method (or a mix of methods), a class schedule, and an instructor that you feel comfortable with. Chances are, the more effort you put into finding a class that's right for you, the more you will get out of it and the better prepared you will be for childbirth.

You might want to begin your search by asking for suggestions from your doctor, from friends who have taken classes, or from your hospital's maternity department. Once you have a list of possibilities, call and ask the instructors to describe their classes and their credentials. You can often learn a lot in a brief phone conversation. It may even be possible to have an interview with the instructor before registering for the class.

Ask about the instructor's qualifications. Is the instructor an employee of a hospital or physicians' group? Does the instructor belong to any local or national organizations of childbirth educators?

Some organizations require their instructors to have a medical background, such as nursing or physical therapy. Others require a college degree in a related field, such as psychology, social work, or education. Some have no special schooling requirements.

Most instructors also receive training in childbirth education. Training may be minimal (for example, the instructor may have been required only to observe a series of classes), or it may be quite rigorous, leading to certification by one of the national or international childbirth organizations. The certification process for these large organizations usually requires classroom sessions or workshops, written work, examinations, observations of childbirth classes, attendance at births, and teaching under supervision.

Ask about the method of childbirth preparation taught in the class. Is it Lamaze, Bradley, Dick-Read, Kitzinger, or a combination of these? Ask, too, about the topics that are covered. Possible topics include self-care in pregnancy, preparation for normal and complicated childbirth, newborn care, breast-feeding and bottle-feeding, and the beginnings of parenthood. You should also find out how much time is actually spent on learning and practicing techniques for coping with labor pain, such as relaxation, breathing patterns,

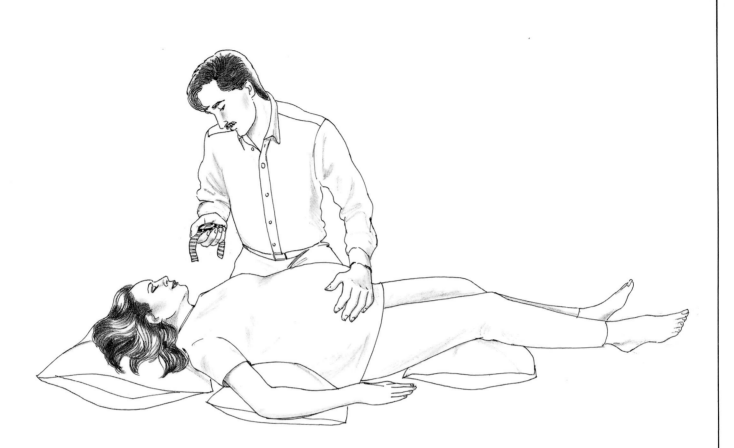

massage techniques, and methods of visualization and focus.

Ask how many actual class sessions are involved. Some classes consist of a series of four sessions, while others consist of as many as 12 meetings. Classes generally meet once a week and may last from one to three hours each time.

How large are the classes? Classes may range in size from private sessions for one or two couples to large classes for 40 to 50 couples. A small, intimate class may be important to you, or you may prefer a more diverse, larger group. If the group is large, does the instructor have one or more trained assistants who can provide more personal contact with the students? Is personal contact with the instructor by phone or by appointment available?

In many communities, specialized classes are also available. Early-pregnancy classes, for example, are generally attended during the first trimester of pregnancy. These sessions cover proper nutrition and exercise, common discomforts of pregnancy and ways to cope with them, development of the baby, and changes that occur in the woman's body in response to pregnancy.

Other specialized classes that may be available in your area include: home-birth classes; refresher classes, for those who had childbirth classes during a previous pregnancy; cesarean-section preparation classes, for those who know that they will have a cesarean section; classes for single mothers, lesbians, parents with a language barrier, parents with impaired

hearing or vision, and teen parents; classes for mothers planning to give their babies up for adoption; classes on vaginal delivery after a previous cesarean section (VBAC); sibling preparation classes for other children in the family; grandparent classes; adoptive parent classes; and breast-feeding classes. Classes for parents after the delivery of the baby are also offered in many communities.

When choosing a childbirth class, you should remember that no childbirth preparation method promises painless childbirth, nor will any method diminish all of the discomforts of pregnancy. The goal of childbirth education is to give couples knowledge and confidence that will enable them to have a positive experience of pregnancy, labor, and delivery.

# Hypertension, Diabetes, and Heart Disease in Pregnancy

The majority of women are healthy at the start of pregnancy and remain so throughout labor and delivery. Aside from experiencing minor discomforts—such as backache, morning sickness, and constipation—most women tolerate well the many physical changes that result from pregnancy.

In some cases, however, a woman may enter pregnancy with a chronic medical problem or may develop a problem during the course of pregnancy. Some of these conditions may affect only the mother, while others may affect both mother and baby.

**Hypertension.** One of the most serious and, unfortunately, most common medical problems in pregnancy is hypertension (high blood pressure). This condition may cause complications in both the mother and the baby. There are two forms of hypertension that may occur in pregnancy: preeclampsia and chronic hypertension.

Preeclampsia (often called toxemia) is a serious condition that develops in the latter weeks of pregnancy. In its most severe form, it is referred to as eclampsia.

The symptoms of this disorder are divided into three stages, each progressively more severe. Mild preeclampsia symptoms include edema (puffiness under the skin due to fluid accumulation in the tissues, usually noted around the face, hands, and ankles), mild elevation of blood pressure, rapid weight gain, and the presence of small amounts of protein in the urine.

Severe preeclampsia symptoms include extreme edema, extreme elevation of blood pressure, the presence of large amounts of protein in the urine, rapid weight gain, headache, dizziness, blurred vision, nausea, vomiting, and severe pain in the upper right portion of the abdomen. Seizures and coma indicate that eclampsia has developed.

The causes of preeclampsia and eclampsia are not known. However, they tend to develop more often in mothers from lower socioeconomic groups and in mothers at the extremes of childbearing age—that is, teenagers and women over the age of 35. One theory proposes that certain dietary deficiencies may be the cause of some cases. Also, there is a possibility that some forms of preeclampsia and eclampsia are the result of a deficiency of blood flow in the uterus.

Preeclampsia and eclampsia cannot be completely cured until the baby is delivered. Before that time, treatment depends, in part, on the severity of the disorder. Mild preeclampsia may be treated with complete bed rest and frequent monitoring. In more severe cases, the woman may be admitted to the hospital so that drugs to control high blood pressure and to prevent seizures can be administered. Drugs may also be given to stimu-

late the kidneys to produce urine. In some severe cases, early delivery of the baby is needed to ensure the survival of both mother and baby.

There is no known way to prevent preeclampsia or eclampsia. Though restriction of salt in the diet may help to reduce swelling, it will not prevent the onset of high blood pressure or the appearance of protein in the urine. During prenatal office visits, the doctor will routinely check weight, blood pressure, and urine. If preeclampsia is detected early, complications for the mother and the baby may be reduced.

Another form of high blood pressure in pregnancy is chronic hypertension. In this condition, high blood pressure usually develops before the fifth month of pregnancy (it may also develop prior to pregnancy). Unlike preeclampsia, there are few if any other symptoms.

Chronic hypertension is more of a threat to the baby than to the mother (and, in general, it is less of a threat than is preeclampsia). Since this condition may cause the placenta to function abnormally, the baby may be affected by a lack of oxygen.

If the hypertension was detected before pregnancy, the doctor may have the woman continue the therapy used to control the disease before pregnancy, as long as it does not involve diuretics or certain types of antihypertensive drugs that can harm the baby. If the high blood pressure developed during pregnancy, antihypertensive drugs may also be used. In either case, both the mother and the fetus will be monitored more closely. Special tests may also be used to determine if the high blood pressure is affecting the baby. If the baby appears to be getting an insufficient supply of oxygen, he will be delivered immediately.

**Diabetes.** Before the discovery of insulin for the treatment of chronic diabetes, women with this disease rarely became pregnant. Today, a diabetic woman can expect to become pregnant and, in most cases, deliver a healthy, normal baby.

Even though medical care for chronic diabetes has greatly improved in the last two decades, the pregnant diabetic is still at increased risk of developing preeclampsia, having a stillbirth, and delivering an abnormally small baby.

For these reasons, a pregnant woman who has chronic diabetes should expect more frequent prenatal office visits and more laboratory testing. It will also be important for her to maintain a strict diet, exercise appropriately, and take her insulin at the prescribed times.

In addition to chronic diabetes, there is a form of diabetes that occurs only during pregnancy. It is called gestational or pregnancy-induced diabetes.

During routine prenatal office visits, a pregnant woman's urine is always tested for the presence of sugar (urine should normally contain no sugar). If sugar is detected in the urine, the doctor will do a series of blood tests to check the woman's blood sugar level and determine if she is suffering from gestational diabetes.

In general, women with gestational diabetes are treated with a special diet that restricts their intake of sugar and carbohydrates. Insulin is rarely necessary

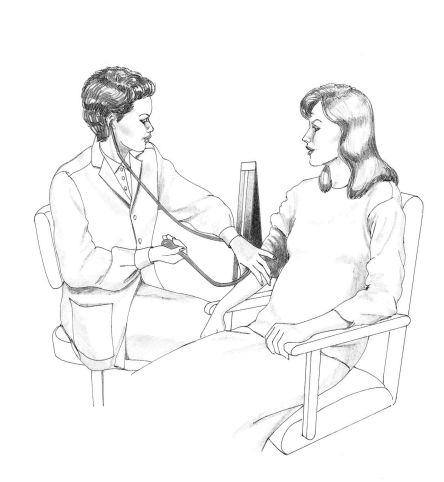

to bring the blood sugar down to normal.

Since the woman with pregnancy-induced diabetes is at a higher risk of developing preeclampsia and having a stillbirth, she can expect to have more frequent prenatal visits and more laboratory testing.

A woman who develops gestational diabetes also has a greater chance of developing true diabetes during her lifetime. For this reason, doctors generally perform another blood sugar test several months after the woman delivers.

**Heart Disease.** Although the incidence of heart disease in women of childbearing age has declined dramatically in recent

years, it still remains one of the major causes of death in pregnant women.

Most women with known heart disease withstand pregnancy without any problems. However, in cases in which the heart muscle or valves are seriously diseased, the added strain that is normally placed on the heart during pregnancy may lead to heart failure and even death.

For this reason, any woman who knows that she has a heart problem should check with her doctor before attempting to become pregnant. A pregnant woman with diagnosed heart disease should expect her pregnancy to be monitored more closely.

# THE THIRD TRIMESTER

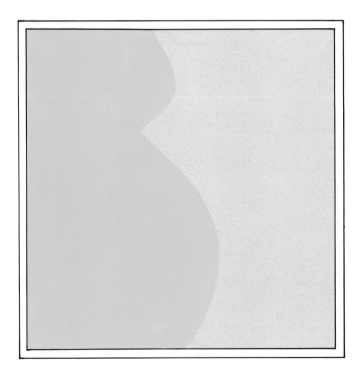

As you enter your last three months of pregnancy, you may find yourself thinking more and more about the upcoming birth. Your large size and your baby's movements are constant reminders that you will become a mother soon.

You may find yourself wanting to slow down a bit, preferring quiet evenings at home, leisurely walks, midday rest breaks, and a generally slower pace to life. The 24-hour-a-day job of making a baby—a job that is nearing completion—becomes tiring in this third trimester.

As your developing baby continues to add weight and strength, you'll want to continue to eat properly, exercise regularly, avoid any possible hazards, and rest up for the work of labor and delivery. Your large size may make many of your usual tasks more difficult and may make getting comfortable seem nearly impossible. But with a little patience and care and a little extra support from those around you, you'll get through your final trimester with flying colors.

As your delivery date draws near, you'll also need to prepare for the arrival of your new baby. You'll need to make room for baby in your home and in your budget. And you'll need to finalize your preparations for labor and delivery.

In the following sections, you'll find discussions of the changes occurring in your baby and in your body in preparation for birth. You'll find strategies for day-to-day living that take into account your changing size and shape. And you'll find practical information about preparing for the big event that's soon to occur.

# THE SEVENTH

# Your Growing Baby

Over the last month, your baby's weight has doubled to between two-and-a-half and three pounds, and she is now about 14 to 17 inches long. She is becoming bigger, stronger, and more able to cope with the world outside your body. With each week that goes by, her chances of living outside your body improve. Even though she is nearly two months away from her expected delivery date, if born now, she could probably survive with the help of intensive medical care.

On the outside, your baby is rapidly filling out her body, but her skin still appears quite wrinkled. Her eyes are open, she has a full head of hair, and her external sexual organs are clearly developed.

Your baby is now even more sensitive to her environment than before. Her eyes can perceive light and objects, her ears can detect sounds both inside and outside

your body, and her skin is highly sensitive to touch, pressure, and pain. Her senses of taste and smell are also highly developed, although she will not need them for several weeks to come.

Internally, numerous changes are taking place that will better prepare your baby to survive outside your body. Within the brain, many new nerve connections are forming that will enable her to react better to her new environment. Her lungs are also maturing.

During the final three months of pregnancy, the baby will gain nearly half of her birth weight, or about three to five pounds. Because of this rapid growth, she needs proper nutrition from you to ensure that she has all of the proteins, minerals, vitamins, and other nutrients necessary to build a strong and healthy body. Poor nutrition at this critical stage of

growth can severely retard her development and may lead to serious problems after birth.

The umbilical cord, which is now about 14 to 18 inches long, forms the lifeline through which

---

**Your baby is over a foot long, her eyes are open, and she has a full head of hair.**

---

the baby receives oxygen and nutrients from your body. For this crucial function, it contains only three blood vessels—two arteries that carry blood from the baby to the placenta, and one vein that brings blood back from the placenta to the baby. The point where the umbilical cord attaches to your baby becomes the umbilicus—more commonly called the navel—after birth.

Inside the umbilical cord is a thick, jellylike substance that surrounds and protects the delicate blood vessels. The firmness of this jelly prevents the blood vessels from being kinked or pinched off if the baby moves around or pushes up against the cord.

Since the umbilical cord is nearly the length of the baby during the last three months of pregnancy, it is possible for it to become tangled around the baby and sometimes even to loop around her neck. This is a common occurrence and usually causes no problems, since the doctor can easily untangle the cord from around the baby during her delivery.

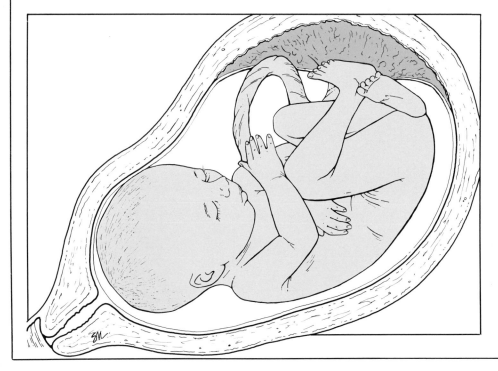

# MONTH

# Your Changing Body

The seventh month marks the start of your last trimester of pregnancy. This is usually considered to be the time of greatest physical discomfort during pregnancy. But this is understandable, since the production of hormones by the placenta is at its highest level, and your uterus—containing baby, placenta, and amniotic fluid—has become quite large and heavy. In addition, the mood swings that you may have experienced earlier in pregnancy have now resumed. With all of this going on, you may be quite ready for your baby to be born.

The new discomforts that you will experience this month are caused mainly by the increasing size and weight of your uterus. Remember that by the seventh month of your pregnancy, you have probably gained at least 15 pounds and your baby now weighs about two-and-a-half to three pounds. This added weight is bound to cause discomfort.

Many women develop varicose veins during the third trimester. As is the case with stretch marks, you are more likely to have varicose veins if your mother or sisters had them during their pregnancies. Varicose veins arise as a result of your uterus pressing against the large blood vessels in your pelvis and abdomen. Since these are the same blood vessels that carry blood from your legs back up to your heart, pressure on them will cause the blood to flow more slowly. As a result, the veins in your legs will become overfilled with blood. As the veins enlarge, they'll be clearly visible through your skin, especially after you have been standing for a long time. The walls of the veins may be stretched to the point

where they will never go back to normal, and you may develop permanent varicose veins.

Hemorrhoids also commonly develop at this stage of pregnancy. Hemorrhoids are enlarged, blood-filled veins in your rectum that, like varicose veins in the legs, result from the pressure of the uterus on blood vessels in the pelvis. In addition, hemorrhoids may

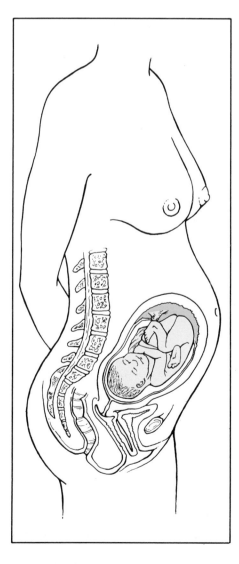

develop as a result of irritation caused by straining when you are constipated. Symptoms of hemorrhoids include painful bowel movements and burning, itching, or pain in the rectal area.

Another change that you may be noticing is swelling of your feet, ankles, and legs. Like hemorrhoids and varicose veins, this swelling results from the uterus pressing on

> You may notice that your feet and ankles will swell if you sit or stand for long periods of time.

blood vessels in the abdomen and pelvis. In this case, however, the swelling is caused by fluid that is forced out of your blood vessels and into the tissues of the legs. Swelling is especially noticeable after you have been standing or sitting for long periods.

During your seventh month, it is also common to develop an aching pain in the groin, vagina, and hips, especially after standing. This, too, may be caused by the uterus pressing on blood vessels in the abdomen and pelvis. Another factor is the stretching of certain bands of tissue, called ligaments, that hold the uterus in place; this so-called "round ligament pain" is often felt in the groin and vagina. In addition, the hormone progesterone causes a loosening of the joints in the pelvis and this may cause pain in the groin and hips.

# How Will I Know When it's Time?

## These descriptions can help you to decide whether or not labor has begun.

Nearly every first-time expectant mother wonders and even worries about whether she'll recognize labor when it begins. You may feel quite helpless, since no conscious action on your part can start labor.

No one really knows exactly what causes labor to begin. As far as we know, it is neither you nor your baby who decides the time of delivery, but rather the placenta and the muscles of the uterus. When conditions are right, the uterus begins contractions that will open the cervix and press the baby down through the birth canal.

How will you know when you are in labor? As basic as this question is, it is often one of the most difficult to answer. It may take hours or even days to figure out whether the sensations you are feeling are labor or something else (prelabor or false labor, for instance). This is because, in most women, labor does not begin suddenly but rather evolves gradually. At some point, you and your doctor will recognize that what you are feeling is true labor.

In this section, you'll find descriptions of prelabor symptoms, false labor symptoms, and signs of labor to help you recognize labor when it begins.

**Prelabor Symptoms (Prodromes of Labor).** As your body is preparing for labor, you may experience the following signs and symptoms, called prodromes of labor. The appearance of these symptoms does not mean that labor will start immediately—it may still be several days before you go into true labor.

*Lightening.* This is the settling or "dropping" of the lowest part of the baby (head or buttocks—whichever is facing downward) into the pelvis. You can often tell that lightening has occurred because the bulge in your abdomen is lower.

As the top of the uterus drops lower, the pressure on your lungs will be relieved and breathing will be easier. At the same time, however, increased pressure on your bladder will cause frequent urination.

If this is your first pregnancy, lightening will probably take place about two to four weeks before labor begins. If you have already had a baby, lightening may not begin until you are in labor.

*Passage of the Mucous Plug ("Bloody Show").* As the cervix begins to dilate (open), the plug of mucus that filled the canal of the cervix is expelled into the vagina. Sometimes, this mucous plug is pink or blood tinged and is commonly called "bloody show."

*Increased Vaginal Secretions.* Your normal vaginal secretions may increase about two weeks before labor.

*The "Nesting Urge."* Many women feel a sudden burst of energy a few days before labor begins. You may feel a nearly uncontrollable urge to scrub floors, prepare the baby's room, clean out closets, straighten cabinets, and do other household work.

*Increased Braxton Hicks Contractions.* During the last month of pregnancy, Braxton Hicks contractions normally increase in frequency and strength. There may be periods in which they become quite strong, making you think that you are in labor. However, Braxton Hicks contractions are usually felt as a "tightening" in the abdomen without much associated pain. Doing something active—walking, for example—usually causes them to stop.

**"False Labor."** Sometimes, a woman will experience what is commonly called "false labor." Although she may be experiencing mildly painful contractions, the pain or discomfort is felt in the lower abdomen rather than in the lower back, and the contractions occur irregularly. Indeed, these false labor contractions, which generally last for less than 30 seconds, may actually start and stop over a period of several days. Also, they usually disappear with activity.

**Labor Sensations.** When labor actually begins, the contractions that labor is beginning (he may, for instance, advise you to call him when the contractions last for at least 30 seconds and have been coming at five-minute intervals for an hour). Do not be afraid to call your doctor if you are unsure. Call the doctor immediately if your bag of waters breaks or leaks, whether or not you have other signs of labor. Make sure that you have your doctor's 24-hour phone number and the phone number of the hospital.

## This Month's Visit

During this month's office visit, your doctor will probably:

- Check your weight. By now, you will have gained about 18 to 20 pounds.
- Check your blood pressure. This will rise slightly to a normal, prepregnancy level.
- Check your urine for sugar and protein. You should still have neither in your urine.
- Ask about symptoms of pregnancy. By now, you may have developed varicose veins, hemorrhoids, swelling of your feet, and pain in the hips and vagina.
- Ask how you are feeling.
- Ask about the baby's movements. The baby's kicking should be noticeable throughout the day.
- Check the growth of your uterus with a tape measure. The top of your uterus should be about two inches higher than it was last month.
- Listen for the baby's heartbeat with a doppler instrument or a stethoscope. The baby's heart should be beating at about 140 to 160 beats per minute.
- Describe what you may feel when you go into labor. He may also arrange for you and your partner to tour the labor and delivery section of the hospital.
- Perform no new blood tests.

are often felt as a cramping pain that begins in the lower back and spreads to the lower abdomen. If you put your hands on your abdomen when you feel this sensation, you will find that your entire uterus is hard.

Generally, labor contractions initially last about 30 to 45 seconds and occur about 15 minutes apart.

Over a period of a few hours, the contractions will become stronger and more painful, they will last longer, and they will occur more frequently. They will not stop with activity like Braxton Hicks contractions do.

During one of your prenatal office visits, ask your doctor when you should call him if you suspect

# Comfort, Rest, and Relaxation

During pregnancy, you need adequate rest because of the added physical and emotional demands that pregnancy puts on your body and your mind. That doesn't necessarily mean that you need to sleep extra hours, but you do need to take short rest breaks throughout each day. During these rest periods, you need to know how to relieve the strain that your changing shape places on your muscles.

The ability to relax is also important, since it allows you to conserve energy, work more productively, and increase your sense of well-being. Being able to consciously relax will also help you during labor, when tension can cause added discomfort.

Before you can get the rest and relaxation you need, however, you need to know how to get comfortable. That's not always an easy task during pregnancy. Fortunately, there are a variety of techniques you can use to increase your comfort throughout pregnancy.

## POSTURE

If you maintain good posture throughout your pregnancy, you will feel more comfortable and you will have more energy. Remember that during pregnancy your posture changes in response to the weight of your enlarging uterus and baby. Many of the minor aches and pains of pregnancy—which can sap your energy and make it difficult to rest—can be reduced if you learn to stand and sit properly. Through correct alignment of your body, you can relieve the strain on

muscles, joints, and ligaments that may prevent you from getting adequate rest and relaxation.

**Standing.** When you are standing, be aware that you will have a tendency to relax your

abdominal muscles and arch your back to compensate for the weight of your uterus. The following techniques will help you to prevent this arching and help you to stand with good body alignment.

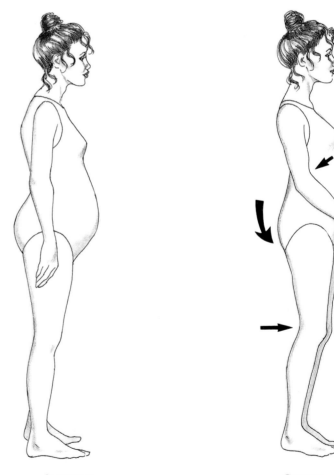

Incorrect                    Correct

*To maintain proper posture, tuck in your chin, tilt your pelvis back, bend your knees and elbows slightly, and keep your feet pointing forward.*

- Tuck in your chin slightly to align your head with your body.
- Tilt your pelvis back by tucking in your abdomen and tightening your buttocks.
- Keep your knees slightly bent and your feet pointed forward, so that the majority of your weight rests on the outer parts of your feet.
- Keep your arms slightly bent.

If you have to stand for a long period of time, place one foot up on a low stool or a step to help prevent your pelvis from tipping forward. If you have to stand with both feet on the floor, shift your weight from one foot to the other or rock back and forth from your heels to your toes to exercise your leg muscles. This will help to force blood back up your legs and help reduce swelling.

**Sitting.** You also need to use proper alignment when you sit, especially if you will be seated for an extended period of time.

- Sit straight up in the chair. Tilt your pelvis back by tucking in your abdomen. Then slide your buttocks slightly forward from the back of the chair so that your lower back comes into contact with the chair back.
- If you need to lean forward—for example, to type or to write at a desk—push your buttocks against the back of the chair and lean your body forward while keeping your back straight.

It may also be helpful while sitting to raise your feet on a low stool. Also, be sure to get up and stretch or walk whenever possible.

## BODY MECHANICS

It is also important during pregnancy to use your body properly and distribute stress evenly to prevent overstretching any one group of muscles or ligaments. By practicing proper body mechanics, you can use your

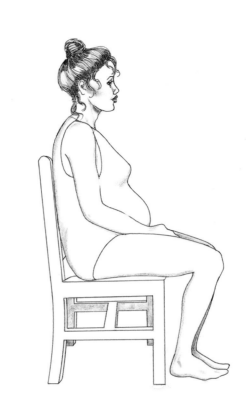

*When resting in a chair, sit straight up, tilt your pelvis back, and slide your buttocks slightly forward from the back of the chair.*

body more efficiently and prevent added strain.

**Reaching Down.** If you need to reach something that is situated on or near the floor, squat down instead of bending over. This way, your leg muscles will do the work of pushing you back into a standing position and you will avoid straining your back muscles. If you need to work over a low table, bend your knees instead of stooping.

**Lifting.** If you need to lift a heavy object, always bring it as close to your body as possible to avoid straining your back. If the object is on the floor, squat down, bring the object close to you, then let your legs push you up. When possible, avoid heavy lifting altogether.

**Climbing Stairs.** Keep your body in good alignment by tipping your pelvis back and keeping your spine straight. This will keep you in proper balance and force your leg muscles to do the work.

**Getting up from Bed.** Roll over on your side. Swing your legs over the side of the bed and use your arms to push yourself into a sitting position. Then rise from the bed using your arms and legs to push yourself up.

**Getting up from the Floor.** Roll yourself onto your side. Using your arms, push yourself to a side-sitting position and then to a kneeling position. Raise one knee and place the foot flat on the floor. Bend over your raised knee, place your hands on the thigh of the raised leg, and push yourself up to a standing position using your arm and leg muscles.

**Getting up from a Chair.** After sliding to the edge of the seat, place one foot slightly in front of the other on the floor. Lean forward and then *push* yourself up off the chair using your arm and leg muscles.

## COMFORTABLE POSITIONS FOR RESTING

Certain positions will make you more comfortable and enhance your ability to rest and relax. These positions will relieve the pressure that your uterus places on various parts of your body and will reduce the strain on muscles, joints, and ligaments.

**Side-Lying.** This is a good position for sleeping and resting; it is also a comfortable position for labor.

Lie on your side with your knees slightly bent. Place pillows between your knees and under your head, shoulders, chest, and abdomen. Move your arms into a comfortable position.

It is always best to lie on your left side, since this moves the weight of the uterus off of the blood vessels in your abdomen and allows excess fluid to drain from your legs.

**Semireclining.** This is a comfortable position for sleeping, resting, watching television, and reading.

Lie in bed or on an armchair. Place pillows under your head, shoulders, and arms to prop yourself up to about a 30 to 40 degree angle.

**Tailor Sitting.** This position will help to shift the weight of the baby and uterus from the back of your pelvis to the front. This is also a very comfortable position during labor.

Sit on a carpet or padded mat with your knees bent and pointing outward. You can let one ankle rest gently on the other, but do not allow one leg to put enough pressure on the other to restrict circulation.

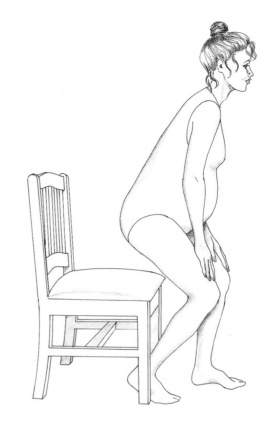

*To get up from a chair, slide to the edge of the chair and place one foot slightly in front of the other on the floor. Lean forward, keeping your back straight, and use your arms and legs to push yourself to a standing position.*

Place soft pillows under your knees for added comfort and let your hands rest gently on your legs.

**Knee-Chest Position.** This is a good position for relieving backache and cramps in the groin and legs.

Get on your hands and knees on a mat, bed, or carpet. Lean forward so that your forearms rest on the ground, and place pillows under your head and chest. Don't stay in this position for more than about two or three minutes.

**Leg Elevation.** This position is useful for decreasing swelling and cramping in the legs.

Prop up your shoulders and back so that you are at about a 30 to 40 degree angle. Raise your legs so that your feet are above the level of your heart. Stay in this position for about three to four minutes.

## RELAXATION

Learning to relax will not only help you to cope with certain discomforts of pregnancy, it will also enable you to conserve strength during labor.

Once you have assumed a comfortable position, you can use any one of a number of methods to relax. Some of these—such as listening to soft music, thinking of a pleasant time and place, or meditating—may already be familiar to you.

To help you consciously relax, pay attention to your breathing and imagine the air passing in and out of your lungs. Tighten the muscles in your body and feel the tension and strain. Then take a deep breath and release the tension. Rest quietly for several minutes and feel the weight and tension leave your body as you relax. Practice relaxation several times a day so that you can become aware of what tension feels like and can learn how to release it.

There are other methods of relaxation that you may find helpful, especially when you are in labor.

**Massage.** Both you and your partner can benefit from massage. Though massage may at times be uncomfortable during labor, it will help you to relieve tension during the latter weeks of pregnancy.

Have your partner use a firm but gentle touch on various muscle groups throughout the body. Practice relaxing your muscles to his touch.

**Touch Relaxation.** To practice touch relaxation, lie down comfortably on pillows and have your partner kneel at your side. Have him gently touch the side of your face. Learn to respond to your partner's touch and to his verbal instruction to "relax" by releasing the tension from your facial muscles. Then, move on to other muscles, such as those in the neck, shoulders, and arms.

Next, have your partner move his hands to either side of your pelvis, low on your hips. Relax your pelvic muscles to his touch. Then, have him move on to your legs and feet.

Practice this exercise every day. Pay attention to the difference between contraction and relaxation of a muscle. Always try to relieve the muscle tension in the direction of your partner's touch.

**Neuromuscular Control Exercises.** During labor contractions, you will need to consciously relax all of your muscles so that your uterus can work freely and efficiently. In order to achieve this, you need to be able to identify

*Tailor Sitting*

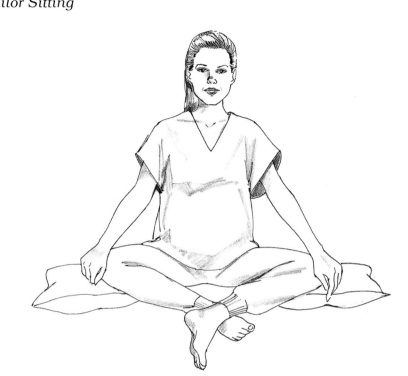

*Tailor sitting is a comfortable position for resting because it shifts the weight of your uterus from the back of your pelvis to the front.*

which of your muscles are contracting and which are relaxing.

To practice this, lie on your back in a comfortable position with all of your joints (knees, elbows, neck, etc.) supported by pillows to ease any strain. Then begin the exercises by contracting your muscles in sequence. Work up from your feet to your neck and face. Next, slowly and consciously relax the same muscles in the same sequence. Pay attention to how the muscles feel as they contract and relax.

Next, try to learn how to contract certain muscles while relaxing all of the others. Begin by contracting the muscles of your right arm while consciously relaxing your left arm and your legs. Then relax your right arm and feel the difference between a muscle that is contracting and one that is relaxing. Then try contracting your left arm and relaxing your right

arm and legs. Do the same with each of your legs.

Once you have contracted and relaxed your arms and legs individually, try contracting your right arm and right leg while relaxing the left side, and vice versa. Each time, concentrate on how the muscles feel when they are contracted and when they are relaxed.

During each exercise, your partner should check the muscles to see which ones are relaxed and which are contracted (the contracted muscles will feel harder). If there is any tension in a muscle that is supposed to be relaxed, spend additional time learning how to relax that muscle group.

Once you have completed this sequence of exercises, remain still and be aware of how your body feels in a state of relaxation. During labor, you should strive for this level of relaxation so that you can let your uterus do all of the work.

# Your Growing Baby

During her eighth month in the womb, your baby will grow to a length of 16 to 18 inches and weigh four-and-a-half to six pounds. Fat is being formed beneath her skin, wrinkles are disappearing, and her body is continuing to fill out. In these last few weeks of pregnancy, she may gain nearly half a pound of weight each week. This is an incredible amount of growth when you stop to think that by the fifth month she weighed only about 12 ounces.

Within your baby's lungs, a substance called surfactant is being formed. Surfactant will prevent the baby's delicate lungs from collapsing when she is born. The lungs are the last organ in your baby's body to mature, and once the lungs are ready, your baby can easily survive outside your body.

The movements of your baby's arms and legs are now much stronger and more coordinated than in previous months because her muscles have grown larger, her bones have hardened, and her nervous system has developed more nerve connections. While once her movements were twitches and flutters, they are now purposeful and graceful. You may actually be able to identify movements of the arms and legs as they push up on the uterus and make small bumps beneath your skin.

Now that the baby has grown to a length of 16 to 18 inches, however, she can no longer move her body around as freely as she could when she was smaller. Soon, by virtue of her size, she will have to stay in one position until birth.

The most common position for your baby to be in during the last two months of pregnancy is the head-first or cephalic position—with her head in the lower part of your uterus and her legs and buttocks up near your chest. At this stage of pregnancy, about 95 percent of babies are in the head-first position.

In some cases, though, the baby may be in the breech position—that is, with her feet and buttocks in the lower part of your uterus and her head up near your chest. About three percent of babies are in the breech position during the last two months of pregnancy. In some cases, your doctor may be able to turn the baby from a breech to a cephalic position within the uterus. A breech baby, however, can be born vaginally as long as the baby's head will fit through the pelvic area. Otherwise, a cesarean section may be performed.

Rarely, your baby may be in the transverse position. Here, instead of the baby lying up and down, she is lying crosswise or perpendicular to your body, with her head on one side of your uterus (for example, to the right) and her legs and buttocks on the other side (for example, to the left). The problem with a baby lying in the transverse position is that she cannot fit through your pelvis and vagina this way. Only one baby in a thousand is in the transverse position at the time of birth. If the position of the baby makes vaginal delivery too dangerous or simply impossible, a cesarean section will generally be performed (see page 100).

It may be possible for you to tell the position of your baby by the force and location of her movements. Since she makes the most powerful movements with her legs, her legs are probably in the area of the abdomen where you feel the most forceful kicks.

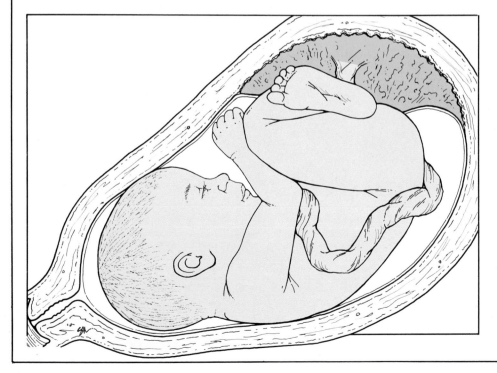

# MONTH

# Your Changing Body

During the eighth month of your pregnancy, your body continues to go through many changes. Now, however, some of these changes are in preparation for the actual birth of your baby. What's more, your uterus is growing even larger, and you may develop new discomforts related to its size.

By now, your uterus will have grown upward into your abdomen to a level just below the bottom of your breast bone. Since the enlarged uterus is now pushing up on your diaphragm (the muscle that separates the chest from the abdomen) and lungs, you may begin to experience shortness of breath, especially when you are sitting or lying down. Climbing stairs or even walking short distances may force you to stop to catch your breath. Bending over may also be a problem, since this position causes the uterus to press even more firmly on your lungs.

You may also find it more difficult to fall asleep, even though you may be very tired. Backache, pressure on your stomach, the movement of the baby, and shortness of breath may all contribute to restless nights.

Many women also begin to experience occasional heart palpitations at this stage of pregnancy. These sensations of rapid heartbeat and fluttering in the chest are not abnormal; they are caused by the increase in heart rate that is needed to supply blood to the baby and placenta. Normally during pregnancy, your heart rate, or pulse, will increase by about ten to 15 beats per minute. So if your normal heartbeat before pregnancy was 75 beats per minute, don't be surprised if your heartbeat now is about 90 beats per minute.

Changes are occurring in your abdomen, too. You may now notice that you are carrying your baby farther in front than you ever did before. It may seem as though your abdomen has sagged and that your uterus is now pointing outward instead of upward. This common change occurs for two reasons.

First, the muscles of your abdomen have weakened from

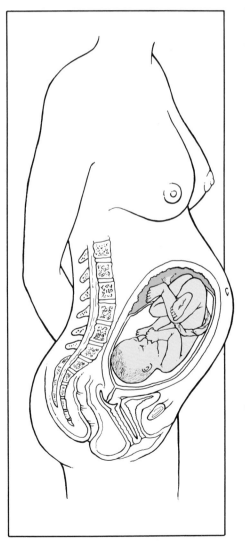

eight months of being stretched by the enlarging uterus. Like a girdle that has lost its elasticity, the abdomen can no longer hold up the weight, so your uterus tends to lean forward.

The second reason is that certain muscles in your abdomen have separated, and the skin between them cannot hold the uterus up. This condition, called diastasis recti, is caused by the separation of the two thick muscular bands that run down the middle of your abdomen from the breast bone to the pubic bone. In some cases, these two muscles, which are normally side-by-side, may actually become separated by three to six inches. If you have had a previous baby, muscle separation and weakness may be even greater and you will carry your baby out in front earlier in pregnancy.

Your body is also undergoing a number of changes that will prepare it for childbirth. The walls of your vagina are becoming more relaxed and the size of the vagina is increasing. This change will make it easier for the baby to pass through the vagina during childbirth. Within a few weeks after delivery, the walls of the vagina will strengthen and contract to decrease the size of the vagina.

Another change that occurs in preparation for childbirth is a loosening and separation of the joints that hold the bones of the pelvis together. This is the body's way of enlarging the space inside your pelvis to make it easier for the baby to pass through during delivery. You may actually be able to feel a separation in your pubic bones of up to one inch simply by placing a finger in the middle of the bone that lies above your vagina.

# What Methods of Pain Relief are Used in Childbirth?

Just as each pregnancy is unique, each labor and delivery is unique, and it is often difficult to determine beforehand if pain relievers will be needed.

The circumstances of your labor and delivery will ultimately affect the types of pain relievers used. The intensity of your contractions, the condition of the baby, the speed of your labor, the type of delivery, and your own tolerance of pain will determine what, if any, drugs are used.

It is important to keep in mind that pain relievers, like other drugs taken in pregnancy, have effects on you and may therefore have effects on your baby. None of the pain-relieving drugs used during childbirth are completely without risk, and, in general, the stronger the drug, the greater the risk of complications.

On the other hand, medical advances have greatly reduced the risks associated with these medications, and there are times during labor and delivery when the

---

> ## You should strive for a safe labor and delivery with a tolerable amount of discomfort.

---

administration of pain relievers is essential for the comfort and safety of mother and baby.

Your primary goal, therefore, should be neither a painless birth nor the refusal of all drugs regardless of the circumstances. Rather,

you should strive for a safe labor and delivery with a tolerable amount of discomfort. Practicing and using various breathing exercises and methods of relaxation (see page 72) can play a vital role in helping you to reach that goal, since they can help make childbirth more comfortable and may decrease the need for pain relievers.

During your prenatal doctor visits, you should ask your doctor about his preferences regarding medication. You should also inform him of your preferences if your labor and delivery are proceeding normally.

**Analgesics.** Analgesics, the mildest form of pain reliever used, decrease the sensation of pain. When used during labor, these drugs are usually injected into a muscle or directly into the bloodstream.

*Levels of Anesthesia*

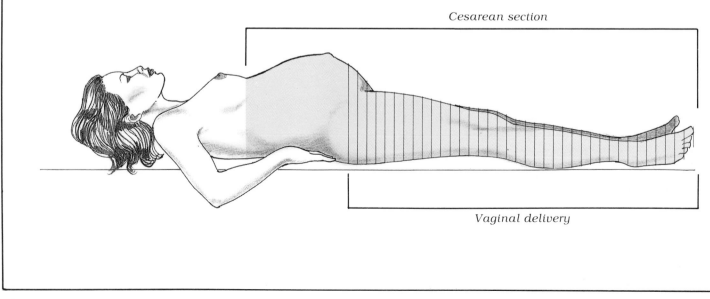

Cesarean section

Vaginal delivery

Morphine and meperidine are the two analgesic drugs most commonly used in obstetrics. Shortly after injection, these drugs will reduce your pain, though you will still be aware of the peaks of your contractions. You may feel nauseated and dizzy shortly after receiving the injection, but these sensations usually pass quickly. Pain relief may last from one to two hours, after which another dose may be given. Analgesics are generally used only in the early and middle stages of labor, since using them nearer to delivery can interfere with the baby's ability to breathe at birth.

**Anesthesia.** Anesthesia means the absence of sensation or feeling. Depending on where they are injected, anesthetic drugs provide varying amounts of pain relief for different lengths of time by causing numbness.

Anesthesia may be either local, regional, or general. In local anesthesia, nerves supplying a certain small area of the body are affected. Three types of local anesthesia are used in childbirth— the paracervical block, the pudendal block, and infiltration of the perineum (the skin and muscles below the vagina).

In the paracervical block, the doctor injects the drug on either side of your cervix, thus blocking pain sensations from the uterus and cervix. The paracervical block is generally used during the later stages of labor or if analgesics are no longer enough to make pain tolerable in earlier stages.

To block pain in the vagina when the baby's head emerges or when an episiotomy is performed (see page 117), an injection into the vagina to block the pudendal nerve may be used. With a pudendal block, you will not feel pain, but you may feel some pressure. Once the anesthesia is injected, it takes about ten to 15 minutes to take effect.

If an episiotomy is necessary and the delivery is progressing too rapidly for a pudendal block to be used, an anesthetic may be injected into the perineum to relieve pain, although pressure and burning will still be felt. This type of anesthesia is not as strong as the pudendal block, but it takes effect much more quickly.

A more powerful form of anesthesia used in childbirth is regional anesthesia. For regional anesthesia, a drug is injected at certain locations that contain nerves supplying large areas of the body. The three forms of regional anesthesia used are the spinal block, the epidural block, and the caudal block. Any of these will cause you to lose all pain from labor and delivery, although you will still feel contractions and pressure.

In the spinal block, a drug is injected directly into the fluid-filled space that surrounds your spinal cord. This effectively blocks all pain from the uterus. By adjusting the amount of drug used and the position of the patient during the injection, the spinal block can also be used to block pain in the abdomen. It can, therefore, be used for either cesarean or vaginal delivery.

The epidural and caudal blocks involve injection of a drug into a space outside the covering of the spinal cord. By adjusting the amount of drug used and the position of the patient when it is injected, the epidural can block pain from the toes all the way to the navel, so it is suitable for either vaginal or cesarean delivery. The epidural can also be used to relieve intense labor pains during the later part of labor, when analgesics can no longer be used and local anesthetics have not proven adequate. The caudal block is generally used only for a vaginal delivery.

General anesthesia, the strongest pain reliever, causes you to lose consciousness. This is usually done through the administration of various gases. General anesthesia is usually used only for emergency cesarean sections or for complicated deliveries when there is an immediate threat to the mother or baby.

## This Month's Visit

During this month's visit, your doctor will probably:

- Check your weight. By now, you will have gained 22 to 24 pounds.
- Check your blood pressure. This should be at your normal prepregnancy level. An elevated level may indicate pre-eclampsia.
- Check your urine for sugar and protein. Protein in your urine may indicate preeclampsia; sugar in your urine may indicate diabetes.
- Ask about symptoms of pregnancy. You may be experiencing shortness of breath and occasional heart palpitations.
- Ask how you are feeling. Report any dizziness, blurred vision, headaches, or swelling of the face and hands, since these may be signs of pre-eclampsia.
- Ask about the baby's movements. The baby should be moving vigorously; if you ever feel that movement is less than usual, inform your doctor immediately.
- Check the growth of your uterus with a tape measure. By the end of this month, the top of your uterus should be just beneath your breastbone.
- Listen for the baby's heartbeat with a doppler or a stethoscope. The baby's heart will now beat about 120 to 160 times per minute.
- Check the position of the baby by feeling the uterus. The baby may either be in the cephalic (head-first), breech (buttocks-first), or transverse (sideways) position.
- Give you a blood test and perform a complete blood count to check for anemia.

# Keeping up the Good Work

Throughout pregnancy, you are confronted with many physical and emotional changes. You may also experience stress caused by your feelings about your changing body and your future role as a parent. During these last three months of your pregnancy, when you're probably just plain tired of being pregnant, it may be encouraging to remember that most of these physical and emotional changes are quite normal and that they'll be quickly overshadowed by the joy you feel when you give birth.

## PRACTICAL MATTERS IN THE THIRD TRIMESTER

As you get ready for the birth of your baby, you will need to continue to be conscientious about your diet and be sure to get plenty of rest. At the same time, however, you'll probably also need to take childbirth preparation classes; make decisions about employment, child care, infant feeding, and health care for your baby; and prepare the baby's space and equipment.

If they have not already done so, this is when most couples take a good look at their financial situation and figure out the impact that the birth of the baby will have. There may be a loss of income for a while, extra bills associated with the birth, other expenses for the baby's needs, and more. It is best to try to prepare yourself for these financial changes as much as possible so that you are not caught in a financial bind when your baby is born.

## COMMON DISCOMFORTS OF THE THIRD TRIMESTER

**Shortness of Breath.** As the uterus continues to enlarge during the last three months of pregnancy, it will push up on your lungs, and you may experience shortness of breath. The best way to relieve this sensation is to maintain an upright position as often as possible and avoid lying flat on your back. The flatter your position, the greater the pressure of the uterus on your lungs.

It may be easy to remain upright during the day, but at bedtime, it will take some preparation. Before you go to sleep, place two pillows under your head and one under your back so that your body is at a slight angle, thus helping to relieve the pressure on your lungs.

If you ever suddenly experience shortness of breath, especially if it is not relieved by standing up or resting, call your doctor, since this could be a sign of a more serious condition such as pneumonia.

**Varicose Veins.** These are common side effects of pregnancy, and they tend to become more severe with each subsequent pregnancy.

Varicose veins are caused by the pressure that the enlarging uterus places on blood vessels in the abdomen that carry blood from the legs back up to the heart. The walls of the veins in the legs weaken as a result of being overfilled with blood. This eventually causes the veins directly below the skin of the legs to bulge and ache.

The following suggestions may help you relieve some of the discomfort of varicose veins and may prevent them from getting worse.

- Elevate your legs on a stool, if possible, while you are sitting.

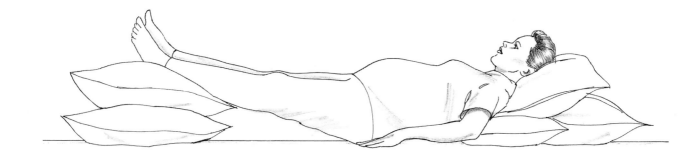

*When resting or sleeping on your back, prop up your chest, shoulders, neck, and head with three pillows to prevent shortness of breath. Raise your feet on pillows or a low stool to prevent blood from pooling in your legs.*

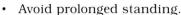
- Avoid prolonged standing.
- Avoid sitting with your knees crossed or sitting in one position for a long period of time.
- If it is possible during the day, take frequent rest periods and lie down with your head and shoulders raised slightly and your feet propped up on a low stool or several pillows.
- Avoid wearing clothing that may constrict the blood vessels in your legs, such as tight slacks, knee-high stockings, or girdles.
- Nonconstricting support stockings may be worn during the day. Be certain to put them on in the morning *before* you get out of bed. If you stand up first, which allows the varicose veins to bulge, the support stockings will be less effective.
- Elevate the foot of your bed with six- to eight-inch blocks. This will raise your legs at night and reduce the pressure on the walls of the leg veins.
- When you are sleeping, lie on your left side. This will help to move the uterus off of the veins in the abdomen and thereby reduce the pressure in the leg veins.

If you ever experience severe pain or tenderness in your legs or notice redness over a leg vein, call your doctor immediately. This may be a sign of a blood clot.

**Dizziness and Light-headedness.** Other problems caused by the pressure of the growing uterus on blood vessels in the abdomen include dizziness and light-headedness. Since this pressure tends to make the blood pool in your legs, less blood is available for your heart to pump up to the brain. These discomforts usually occur if you rise suddenly from a sitting or reclining position, because the heart cannot compensate quickly enough for your new position. Until the heart can compensate by pumping harder, you may experience dizziness and a sensation of light-headedness.

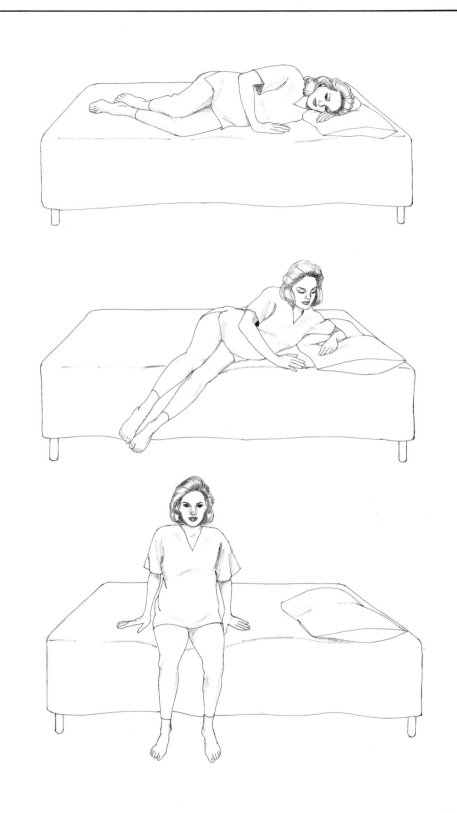

*To prevent dizziness as you rise from bed, roll over onto your side near the edge of the bed. Use your arms to push yourself slowly to a sitting position as you swing your legs over the side of the bed. Remain seated for a minute or two, then slowly push yourself to a standing position.*

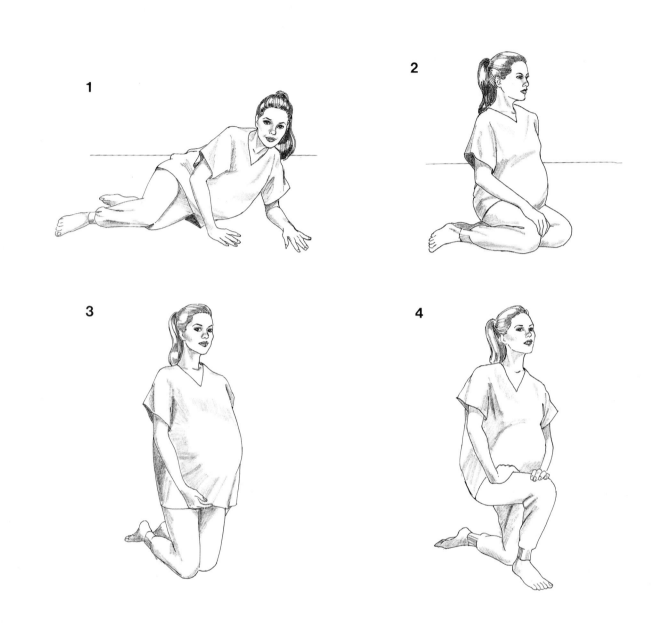

1

2

3

4

*To get up from the floor, roll onto your side and use your arms to push yourself into a side-sitting position and then to a kneeling position. Raise one knee and place your foot flat on the floor. Bend over the raised knee, place your hands on your thigh, and push yourself to a standing position.*

To prevent this from happening, make certain that you avoid sudden changes in your position. Stand or sit up slowly. For example, when you rise from bed in the morning, use your arms to push yourself up slowly to a sitting position. Remain seated for a minute or two, and then slowly stand up.

A low blood sugar level—called hypoglycemia—may also cause dizziness. Since the baby is constantly taking sugar from your blood, your blood sugar level may drop at certain times of the day, usually between meals. To relieve this, always carry a high-carbohydrate snack, such as crackers or an apple. At the first sign of light-

headedness, eat the snack. This will usually relieve symptoms within a few minutes. You may also want to eat several smaller meals throughout the day instead of three large meals, since this will also help to keep your blood sugar level from dropping too low.

**Hemorrhoids.** This problem is also caused by the pressure that the enlarging uterus puts on the veins in the abdomen. The following suggestions may help you relieve hemorrhoids.

- First, try to relieve any constipation (see page 28), since straining to have a bowel movement may cause hemorrhoids to develop and will make existing ones larger.
- Avoid prolonged standing and sitting. Lie down whenever you can.
- For relief, place witch-hazel pads, which you can purchase at a drugstore, directly on the hemorrhoids. You may do this three or four times a day as needed.
- Soak in a warm bath whenever possible.

If these simple measures fail to bring relief, your doctor can prescribe safe medications, such as stool softeners and pain-relieving hemorrhoid creams and suppositories, for you to use.

If extreme pain develops in the rectal area or if you experience any rectal bleeding, notify your doctor.

**Swelling of the Legs, Feet, and Ankles.** This common problem is also caused by the heavy weight of the uterus pressing on blood vessels in the abdomen. It is usually most apparent after you have been standing or sitting for a long period of time.

The following suggestions may help you relieve this swelling.

- Try to lie down or sit with your feet elevated as often as possible.
- Do not wear constricting stockings, panties, or girdles.
- Sleep on your left side with your feet slightly elevated on pillows. This will help to move the uterus off the blood vessels in the abdomen and will aid circulation in the legs.
- Salt in your diet may cause you to retain fluid, which will contribute to swelling. While you should not severely restrict your

salt intake, you may want to avoid heavily salted foods. You might also try cutting back on the use of salt at the table if you add salt while cooking. Consult your doctor if you have any questions about salt in your diet.

While swelling of the legs is common during pregnancy, swelling of the hands or face may be a sign of preeclampsia. If you ever experience swelling of the

---

## Notify your doctor immediately if you develop blurred or double vision during pregnancy.

---

hands or face, or if your feet, ankles, or legs swell suddenly, notify your doctor immediately.

**Aches in the Vagina, Groin, and Hips.** These discomforts are caused by the pressure of the enlarging uterus and the loosening of the joints and ligaments in the pelvis caused by your changing hormone levels.

The best remedy is to avoid activities that may strain these joints and ligaments. Move carefully and avoid sudden twisting or bending. Also, turn over slowly when you are in bed or getting up. Practicing the pelvic tilt exercise (see page 54) may also help to relieve these discomforts.

**Vision Problems.** Women who wear glasses or contact lenses may find that their vision during pregnancy is not as good as it was prior to pregnancy. Vision changes may occur if the shape of the eyeball changes slightly due to increased fluid in the tissues. (Some women experience similar vision changes five to seven days before their menstrual period when they are not pregnant.) If you do have this problem, it may be necessary to have your lens prescription

changed during pregnancy. Talk to your eye doctor about this.

Be sure to notify your doctor immediately if you experience blurred or double vision, since these may be signs of preeclampsia.

## PSYCHOLOGICAL CHANGES

The third trimester is a time of anticipation. Soon, your baby will be born. During these final months of pregnancy, the baby will begin to take on an identity of her own. This is usually when parents-to-be set up the nursery and discuss names for their child.

Usually, by the time the third trimester has arrived, any ambivalent feelings about the pregnancy have been resolved. During this time, you may feel very special. If you had difficulty becoming pregnant in the first place, the last weeks of pregnancy may take on even more significance.

During this time, you may find that you need extra attention from your husband, your family, and your friends. You may need reassurance regarding your appearance and your ability to be a good parent.

First-time mothers often experience a great deal of anxiety at this time about whether they will know when labor has begun. In women who have had children before, Braxton Hicks contractions may be so strong that they may not know when real labor has started. Childbirth classes, which are usually attended in the seventh or eighth month of pregnancy, are very helpful in educating parents-to-be about what they can expect and in relieving many common fears about childbirth.

For your husband, impending fatherhood may trigger memories and emotions concerning his childhood relationship with his own father. For some men, becoming a father means giving up the idea of being a son. It also means reconciling childhood experiences with the reality of becoming a father. In some men, it seems that these feelings are stronger during the latter weeks of pregnancy than they are after birth.

Even if a man has fathered children before, his wife's pregnancy may elicit a variety of emotions and thoughts. He may think about the kind of father he has been to the children that he has, and he may worry about the additional responsibilities he will be facing. If the father-to-be is proud of his fathering experience, he will probably be excited about the upcoming birth.

Just as it was assumed in the 1950s that no father could adequately participate in the labor and delivery experience, it is now assumed that most fathers will. If your husband plans to attend the birth, he may be concerned about his ability to act as your coach during labor, especially if this is your first baby. Talking to other men who have gone through the experience may be helpful. Often, childbirth preparation classes provide the perfect opportunity for this type of discussion.

If your husband feels that he will not be able to participate in labor and delivery, this should be discussed and resolved prior to the event. You and your husband should not feel that this decision is in any way wrong or abnormal.

It is very important during the third trimester for you and your husband to communicate your needs, fears, and concerns openly and to provide each other with support and reassurance. Childbirth preparation classes can also be a great source of reassurance and will increase your knowledge and decrease your fears about the events ahead. You may find it comforting to be able to talk to other couples and may find that they share many of the same emotions and concerns.

## SEXUAL RELATIONS

How couples feel about sexual relations during the last few

months of pregnancy varies greatly. Some couples may experience a renewal of the romantic bond that may have been missing during the previous few months. However, other couples may have a decline in sexual interest and may limit their sexual activity.

Some women feel quite self-conscious about their bodies during the last months of pregnancy. A large abdomen, swollen

---

> It is important to have realistic expectations about what your life will be like after your baby is born.

---

breasts, increased vaginal secretions, and increased skin pigmentation may cause a woman to feel unattractive and even embarrassed. This can affect her relationship with her husband. On the other hand, some women may feel that these changes enhance their sexuality, and they may have an increased desire for sex.

Men, too, will have feelings about their partner's changing body. Some men will take great delight in feeling the baby's movements and massaging the abdomen. Others, however, may be uncomfortable with their partner's physical appearance or may fear that they will hurt the baby during sexual intercourse.

During the last few months of a normal pregnancy, sexual intercourse poses little threat of infection to the baby as long as the amniotic sac has not ruptured. Orgasm can initiate labor contractions only if the woman is near her due date. The erect penis will not hurt the baby and is unlikely to rupture the amniotic sac.

If you have developed any complications during your current

pregnancy or if you experienced complications in a previous pregnancy, however, be sure to discuss with your doctor any limits that might be placed on sexual activity. Likewise, if you have any concerns about safe sexual activity during pregnancy, consult your doctor.

It is important that you communicate with your partner and discuss how you feel about sexual relations. Your increasing size may necessitate some experimentation with positions for intercourse. You may, for example, want to try intercourse lying side by side or with you on top. The important point is to find a position that is comfortable for both of you and that does not place too much stress on your body.

If having intercourse during these last months of pregnancy makes either of you uncomfortable or if your doctor has advised that you abstain for medical reasons, keep in mind that there are other ways of expressing your love for one another, such as touching, kissing, and cuddling.

For many couples expecting their first child, the impending birth may make them acutely aware that they will never be simply a couple again—they will also be parents. This may lead to fears that they will be unable to experience the intimacy that they enjoyed before the baby. Other parents-to-be try to convince themselves that life will be unchanged after their child is born. Neither view is realistic.

The birth of a child will bring with it multiple changes, both in the couple's relationship and in their daily activities and plans. It is critical that expectant parents discuss these issues before the birth of their child. Expectant parents who have convinced themselves that nothing will change will be in for a great many disappointments and frustrations. The idea that they are in control of so profound an experience will be a disappointing fantasy once the

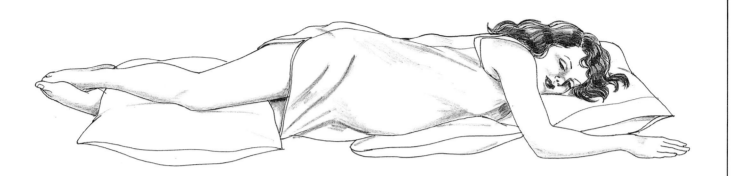

*For a comfortable night's sleep, lie on your left side with your knees slightly bent. Place pillows between your knees and under your head, shoulders, chest, and abdomen.*

baby is brought home from the hospital.

On the other hand, those who have realistic expectations about the pregnancy and about life with a newborn will be more likely to cope well and perhaps even enjoy many of the changes.

## SAFEGUARDING YOUR BABY'S HEALTH

During the third trimester, your baby remains vulnerable to the effects of drugs, toxic chemicals, radiation, and infection. Since this is also a time of rapid growth, your baby may be severely affected by any nutritional deficiencies in your diet.

Even though she is protected by the amniotic fluid and your abdominal wall, your baby can still be injured if you have an accident in which you suffer trauma to the abdomen. Rupture of the membranes, separation of the placenta from the wall of the uterus, and even physical injury to the baby can occur if you have a serious accident.

For these reasons, you need to be especially careful during the third trimester to avoid situations in which there is potential for injury. For example, you may wish to stop driving a car if your enlarged

abdomen has made it difficult for you to maneuver the steering wheel or reach the pedals. You should avoid standing on ladders or chairs, since you may easily lose your balance and fall. You should also avoid any sporting activity in which you may either lose your balance or get hit by a ball or a teammate.

It is also important that you keep in mind the signs and symptoms that may indicate that a problem is developing in your pregnancy (see p. 58). If you ever feel that you are developing any of these signs, call your doctor immediately.

## FOR YOUR COMFORT

**Sleep.** During the last few months of your pregnancy, you may find it difficult to find a comfortable position for sleeping. Many factors contribute to this, including shortness of breath, leg cramps, backache, movement of the baby, and the large size of your abdomen.

You may sleep in any position that you find comfortable, since it is not possible for you to harm the baby by compressing or rolling onto your uterus. The use of several pillows positioned beneath your head and back and between your

legs may help you to get comfortable. If you are experiencing shortness of breath, you may wish to use more pillows under your head and back so that you are in a semireclining position. A heating pad or hot-water bottle under your back or legs may also be helpful.

Never use sleeping pills during pregnancy, since their effects on the baby are not entirely known. A short walk in the open air, a glass of warm milk, or a warm shower or bath will often help to relieve insomnia.

**Exercise.** During the last few weeks of pregnancy, it is best to avoid most forms of strenuous exercise, including jogging and tennis, since you will become out of breath easily and your balance may be affected by the size and weight of your uterus.

Walking and swimming remain excellent forms of exercise during the latter months of pregnancy, since they are safe activities, and they will help maintain good circulation in your legs and good muscle tone in your legs and abdomen.

**Travel.** During the last month of pregnancy, it is best to travel no farther than one hour's distance from the hospital in which you intend to deliver.

# Will I Need a Cesarean Section?

## If a serious complication arises during your labor, a cesarean section may be necessary to ensure the health and safety of both you and your baby.

While the majority of babies born in the United States are delivered vaginally, about 15 to 20 percent are delivered by cesarean section. Cesarean section is the delivery of a baby by cutting through the mother's abdominal wall and uterus and removing the baby from the mother's body through these incisions.

A cesarean section may be performed for many reasons. In general, a cesarean section is performed when a vaginal delivery would cause injury to either the mother or the baby. For example, a cesarean section may be performed in order to:

- Save the baby's life when a problem with the placenta or the umbilical cord is cutting off the blood supply to the baby. An abnormal heart rate in the baby, which is usually detected with a fetal monitor (see page 113), may indicate that such a problem has developed.
- Deliver the baby if the mother fails to give birth vaginally after a long labor. This usually occurs because the baby is simply too big to pass through the mother's pelvis.
- Prevent infection of the baby when dangerous bacteria are present in the amniotic fluid or

### Today, cesarean section is a very safe operation.

when a potentially dangerous vaginal or cervical infection, such as herpes, is present in the mother.
- Prevent injury to the baby during a breech birth (when the baby would emerge through the vagina with her buttocks or feet first rather than in the usual head-first position). Many obstetricians believe that all breech births in first-time mothers and all premature breech births should be done by cesarean section.
- Treat a disease or condition in the mother or baby that can be treated more successfully if birth occurs as soon as possible.

- Prevent the possibility that the uterus may rupture during labor in a woman who had a cesarean section with a previous baby.
- Deliver three or more babies in a multiple pregnancy.

There are two types of cesarean section, each used for a particular reason. In the classic cesarean section, the doctor makes a vertical incision in the mother's abdomen from her navel to her pubic bone; the thick upper portion of the uterus, which lies beneath the skin of the upper abdomen, is also cut vertically down the center.

The classic cesarean section is generally used only if the baby is lying in an abnormal position or if the placenta is in an abnormally low position in the uterus (placenta previa). With this type of cesarean section, there is more bleeding than with other methods, it is more difficult for the doctor to repair the incision, and the uterus is more likely to rupture during a future pregnancy. For these reasons, the classic cesarean section is seldom used today unless absolutely necessary.

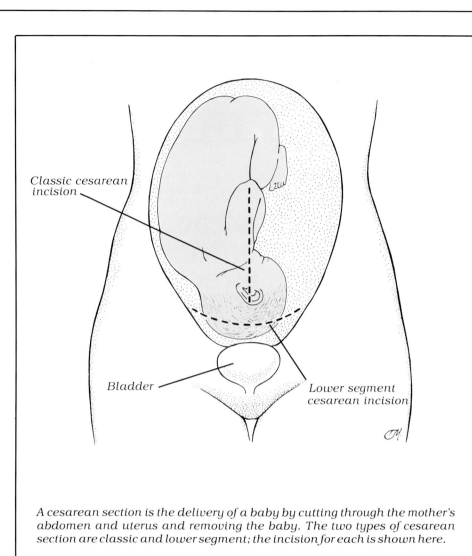

*Classic cesarean incision*

*Bladder*

*Lower segment cesarean incision*

*A cesarean section is the delivery of a baby by cutting through the mother's abdomen and uterus and removing the baby. The two types of cesarean section are classic and lower segment; the incision for each is shown here.*

having a cesarean section, you should keep in mind that if a serious complication arises during labor, a cesarean section may be necessary to ensure the health and safety of both you and your baby.

## This Month's Visit

During this month's office visit, your doctor will probably:

- Check your weight. By now, you will have gained about 22 to 28 pounds.
- Check your blood pressure. Your blood pressure should remain normal. If it is elevated, you may be developing pre-eclampsia.
- Ask about symptoms of pregnancy. By now, you may have experienced lightening, an increase in vaginal discharge, passage of the mucous plug, and an increase in the frequency of Braxton Hicks contractions.
- Ask how you are feeling. Be certain to report any dizziness, blurred vision, headaches, or swelling of the face and hands, since these may be signs of preeclampsia.
- Ask about the baby's movements. The baby should be moving vigorously; if you ever feel that your baby is moving less than usual, inform your doctor immediately.
- Check the growth of your uterus with a tape measure. Since the baby may have dropped lower in your uterus, the top of the uterus itself may now be a few inches below your breastbone.
- Listen for the baby's heartbeat with a doppler instrument or a stethoscope. The baby's heart will now beat about 120 to 140 times per minute.
- Check the position of the baby by feeling the uterus.
- Do a pelvic examination to check if the cervix is dilating (opening) or effacing (thinning out).
- Perform no new tests.

The lower segment cesarean section is the more commonly performed operation. Here, the doctor makes an incision—either vertically or in a smile-shape— through the lower part of the abdomen and the lower, thinner portion of the uterus.

In the past, a firm rule in obstetrics was "once a section, always a section," because of the fear that the uterus would rupture if a vaginal delivery were attempted in a subsequent pregnancy. More recently, however, obstetricians have found that many women who have had a previous cesarean section can have a safe vaginal delivery in a subsequent pregnancy.

If you have already had a baby by cesarean section, you may want to ask your doctor if it is possible for you to attempt a vaginal delivery.

Sometimes, it is necessary for a cesarean section to be performed before a woman actually goes into labor. In most cases, however, the doctor does not know if a cesarean section will be needed until the woman is in labor. There is really nothing that you can do before labor to prevent the need for a cesarean section.

Today, cesarean section is an extremely safe operation because of improved antibiotics and better anesthetic medications. While you may not relish the thought of

# THE THIRD TRIMESTER: PLANNING AND PREPARATION

instead of rushing through it when you are in labor? What type of insurance forms should you bring? Remember, it is a lot easier to ask these questions now than it will be when you are in labor.

Questions about hospital procedures and policies need to be asked carefully. For example, if you ask "What usually happens to the baby after he or she is born?" you will probably learn more than if you ask "What is the hospital's procedure for routine newborn care?" Some hospitals may not have specific policies, but they will have customs, and these are what you will want to know.

You might ask for a step-by-step description of what happens after a woman in labor arrives. Do most women have a nurse assigned to them, or do the nurses take care of more than one laboring woman at a time? Is it customary for women

to receive pain medications, or do most women use little or no pain medication? If a woman desires a natural or unmedicated childbirth, is she actively encouraged and supported in this by the staff? What types of pain medication and anesthesia are available? Is there an anesthesiologist (a doctor who specializes in administering anesthesia) in the hospital at all times or is he called in only when needed? Is a pediatrician in the hospital at all times, or is he called in only when needed? Do most women receive intravenous fluids and continuous electronic fetal monitoring (see page 113)? How long is the usual hospital stay? You may want to find out if there's a "short stay" program that allows mothers and babies to go home within a few hours after birth.

Finally, during your hospital tour, clarify the costs of labor and

delivery rooms, nursery charges, and so forth. You might be surprised at how hospitals, even those in the same town or area, may vary in their charges. You will also want to check your insurance policy to determine how much you may need to pay out of your own pocket.

**Out-of-Hospital Birth.** Out-of-hospital birth is an option only for the healthy woman who is experiencing a normal pregnancy and who has never experienced complications in any previous pregnancies. A woman who is experiencing a complicated pregnancy or who may require a cesarean section will need to labor and deliver in a hospital that is equipped to handle these situations. If you are considering an out-of-hospital birth, it is extremely important to keep in mind that emergencies can develop rapidly and often without warning during labor and delivery. Most out-of-hospital settings will not have the medications and equipment that may be necessary in an emergency.

If out-of-hospital birth is an option for you, you will need to find out what services are available in your community. Many cities now have birthing centers. These are freestanding facilities that are staffed by medical professionals. Birthing centers offer an alternative to hospital birth for the healthy pregnant woman who is not at increased risk of experiencing a complicated birth (many of these centers will not accept women who have a greater likelihood of needing a cesarean section or other type of sophisticated medical intervention).

These centers attempt to offer "the best of both worlds" by providing family-centered care in a homelike setting but with the security and safety provided by a professional staff, up-to-date monitoring equipment, and prearranged emergency backup. These centers can deal with normal pregnancies, and they may have the equipment necessary to detect

---

## Packing Your Suitcase

The following are some items that you may want to take with you to the hospital when you go into labor. Pack your bags at least two weeks before your due date so that you do not have to rush around at the last minute.

### For the mother during labor:
- Massage oil (not lotion) or powder (cornstarch is best)
- Toothbrush and toothpaste
- Lip balm
- Rolling pin, tennis balls, or other massage aids
- Hot-water bottle or plastic ice pack for comfort
- Juice, ice pops, or sour-candy suckers
- Music tapes and a battery-operated tape machine
- Cotton socks
- Hair clips or rubber bands
- Breath spray

### For the father:
- Food/snacks
- Breath mints or toothbrush
- Camera and film

- Watch with a second hand for timing contractions
- Pencil and paper

### For the baby:
- Warm hat (may be provided by the hospital)
- Stretch suit or T-shirt, receiving blanket, warm blanket and booties (depending on weather), and four or five diapers for taking baby home
- Car seat

### For the mother after birth:
- Nursing bras (two or three)
- Nursing pads
- Breast cream or lotion
- Personal hygiene items, cosmetics, and a shower cap
- Phone numbers of people to call with the good news
- Reading and writing materials, birth announcements, stamps, address book
- Comfortable clothes to wear home (stick with adjustable or loose-fitting clothing so that it's sure to fit)

---

complications that may develop. They may not, however, have the equipment or staff necessary to deal with such complications. A pregnant woman who experiences an unexpected complication will be transferred immediately to a hospital that is equipped to handle the problem.

Before you consider using a birthing center, make certain that it is licensed by the state. You should also check with your insurance company to be sure that your policy covers childbirth in a freestanding birthing center.

Another alternative to traditional hospitals is home birth. During the last two decades, the number of home births in the United States has greatly increased, as parents have attempted to make

childbirth a more personal and family-oriented experience. The delivery is performed by either a doctor or a midwife and generally takes place in the family's bedroom.

Medical intervention is often not necessary for a healthy woman who is experiencing a normal labor. During a home birth, a woman who does develop an unexpected complication must be transferred to a hospital immediately. This disadvantage of out-of-hospital birth should be carefully considered by all women planning birth outside the hospital.

When inquiring about out-of-hospital birth services, find out what drugs and equipment are generally used. Are intravenous fluids, pain medications, or fetal monitors used? What emergency

equipment is on hand for every birth?

You will also need to know what hospital is used in case a transfer becomes necessary. Who makes the transfer arrangements? Is an ambulance readily available? How far away is the backup hospital?

Out-of-hospital birth offers parents certain advantages and experiences that they may not have with a traditional hospital birth. They have more control over birth procedures and there are few routines that need to be followed. Contact with the baby after birth is limited only by the parents' wishes. When considering these advantages, however, you must weigh them carefully against the risks to both mother and baby if an emergency should occur.

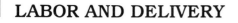

insert two gloved fingers into the opening of your cervix; the distance that the fingers can be spread apart is then judged. If your doctor says that your cervix is dilated to four centimeters, this means that you have six centimeters to go until the cervix is completely open (ten centimeters). In medical terms, the word "complete" means that your cervix is completely thinned out (100 percent effaced), and completely dilated (ten centimeters in diameter).

## FACTORS THAT INFLUENCE YOUR LABOR

The length and difficulty of labor vary from woman to woman, and even from pregnancy to pregnancy in the same woman. Some labors are very fast, lasting only a few hours. Some are average in length, lasting about 15 to 16 hours for first-time mothers and about seven to eight hours for women who have had babies before. Some are very long, lasting nearly a day. Some labors start slowly and then speed up unexpectedly. Others start rapidly and then slow down. The amounts of pain and fatigue vary also.

Many factors play a part in how long and how difficult your labor will be. You can influence some of these factors, but not others. Factors you cannot control include:

- The size and shape of your pelvic bones
- The size and shape of the baby's head and shoulders
- The condition of your cervix when labor begins
- The strength of your contractions
- The position of the baby
- Some aspects of your general health and your baby's well-being

Factors that you can control, to some extent, include:

- Your emotional state and attitude toward birth (whether you are anxious and tense or relaxed and confident)
- The presence of a helpful, caring partner
- Knowledge of what to expect
- An environment and professional staff that help you feel secure
- Good prenatal care (including good nutrition and good health habits)

The length of your labor and your success in delivering the baby vaginally will be influenced most by

---

## Your baby's size will help determine how quickly labor progresses.

---

the strength and coordination of your uterine contractions, the size and position of the baby, and the size and shape of your pelvic bones.

**Your Contractions.** The strength and coordination of your contractions play major roles in determining the progress of your labor, because the contractions open your cervix and push the baby down. In general, the more powerful, coordinated, and frequent your contractions, the more quickly and efficiently labor will progress. If labor is progressing very slowly, your doctor may ask you to walk around to help stimulate contractions. If necessary, a drug may be administered to speed the process along.

**Size of Your Baby.** In addition to the strength and coordination of your contractions, the size of your baby will play a major role in determining how quickly your labor progresses and how successful you are at delivering your baby vaginally. Since the baby must pass out of your body through the rigid walls of your pelvis, his size is

important if he is to fit through safely. If he is too large to pass through, a cesarean section will be necessary. Even with the aid of techniques such as ultrasound, it is difficult to predict the size of the baby before labor begins.

**Presentation.** Presentation refers to which end of the baby is closest to your cervix. In about 97 percent of pregnancies, the baby presents in a head-first or cephalic position. That is, his head is in the lower part of the uterus and his buttocks are at the top of the uterus near the mother's chest. In about two-and-a-half percent of pregnancies, the baby is in a breech presentation, meaning that his buttocks are in the lower part of the uterus and his head is at the top. Rarely, the baby may present in a transverse position, meaning that he is lying sideways and that one of his shoulders is in the lower part of the uterus. In general, the baby's head is the part that most effectively dilates the cervix. Therefore, labor is likely to progress more smoothly if the baby is in a head-first position during his final weeks in the uterus.

**Position.** Your baby's position will also affect your labor. Position refers to the direction that the baby is facing in relation to your back. He may be facing your back, facing away from your back, or facing sideways. Labor and delivery are usually least painful and more rapid if the baby is facing your back.

**Size and Shape of Your Pelvis.** The third factor that will influence your labor is your pelvis. Your baby must pass through the cavity surrounded by your pelvic bones to reach the outside world. During your first prenatal visit, your doctor probably determined the size and shape of your pelvic opening when she performed a pelvic examination. If the opening of the pelvic cavity is too small or if it has an unusual shape, even an average-sized baby may not be able to pass through it safely. If this is the case, a cesarean section will be required.

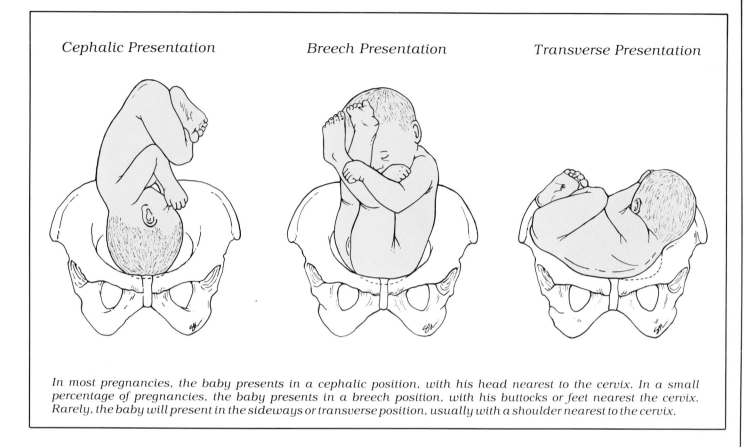

Cephalic Presentation    Breech Presentation    Transverse Presentation

*In most pregnancies, the baby presents in a cephalic position, with his head nearest to the cervix. In a small percentage of pregnancies, the baby presents in a breech position, with his buttocks or feet nearest the cervix. Rarely, the baby will present in the sideways or transverse position, usually with a shoulder nearest to the cervix.*

## THE STAGES OF LABOR

Labor is described as having four stages. The first stage begins with the onset of true labor contractions and lasts until your cervix is completely dilated. The second stage begins when your cervix is completely dilated and ends when your baby is born. *Delivery of your baby, therefore, occurs during the second stage of labor.* The third stage begins after your baby is delivered and ends when the placenta is expelled. The fourth and final stage begins once the placenta is expelled and lasts until your medical condition has stabilized.

**The First Stage.** The first stage is almost always the longest (lasting anywhere from two to 24 hours or more). It usually starts slowly and then speeds up when the dilation of the cervix reaches about four to five centimeters. Your contractions may not be clear and strong at first, but they will become longer, stronger, and closer together with time.

Much of your time in the first stage of labor may actually be spent trying to figure out if you are in labor or not. If you can be distracted from your contractions, it is unlikely that you are in very advanced labor.

**Determining that labor has begun.** If you are in the latter half of your pregnancy, you probably have already felt your abdomen getting hard and then relaxing and getting soft. Perhaps you have also experienced menstrual-like cramping in the lower part of your abdomen near your pubic bone. These are all contractions, but they do not indicate that you are in labor. Unlike true labor pains, these so-called Braxton Hicks contractions are usually more uncomfortable than painful and they usually occur irregularly and in different areas of the uterus. They serve to soften, thin out, and slightly dilate the cervix before you actually go into labor. During the third trimester, these contractions will get stronger.

Once labor begins, your contractions will start at the top of your uterus and then spread down toward the cervix in a regular, rhythmic pattern. In this way, the baby will be pushed downward in the direction of the vagina with each contraction.

Each labor contraction has three parts that you will easily feel: the gradual buildup; the peak or apex; and the tapering off. Between each contraction, there will be a relaxation period during which the uterus rests and no contraction occurs. The next contraction will begin in the same fashion, by building up, peaking, and then tapering off into relaxation.

Timing your contractions will help you to know when you are in labor and how your labor is progressing. When you think you are in labor and you call the doctor or hospital, you will be asked to describe your contractions in terms of duration, frequency, interval, and intensity.

- The duration of a contraction is measured from the time that you first feel it to the first moment that the uterus is completely relaxed.
- The frequency of contractions is measured from the beginning of one contraction to the beginning of the next.
- The interval is the time between the end of one contraction and the start of the next.
- The intensity of a contraction is an observation that only you can make. You will need to compare the strength of the latest contractions with the strength of previous ones.

Remember that the contractions you will feel in early labor will be just the beginning, and there is normally no need to rush to the hospital after your first two strong contractions. You'll probably have to wait several hours before it will be time to go to the hospital. As labor progresses, a pattern will develop in which your contractions will become stronger, longer, more painful, and closer together; there will be little if any doubt that you are in labor.

**False labor.** Sometimes women will experience what is often called "false labor." This is not really "false," but rather a period when contractions are generally irregular and the cervix is not dilating. These contractions may actually start up and stop over several days. The chart above shows some differences between true labor contractions and "false labor" contractions and may help you to decide if you are in labor. Remember that you may not always

## Contraction Chart

| CONTRACTION CHARACTERISTIC | True Labor | False Labor |
|---|---|---|
| Duration | Contractions gradually increase in length | No change, length irregular |
| Interval | Rest periods between contractions gradually become shorter | No change, length of rest period irregular |
| Frequency | Contractions come closer and closer together with time | No change, occur irregularly |
| Intensity | Gradually become stronger | No change, intensity varies |
| Location | Back and abdomen | Abdomen only, starting in no particular location |
| Effect of mother's activity | Continue regardless | Will slow down or stop with walking or lying down |

follow a "textbook" pattern. If you are unsure if labor has begun, call your doctor, or go to the hospital, where a nurse can check you.

**When to call the doctor.** During your prenatal visits, you should ask your doctor when she wants you to report labor to her and when you should go to the hospital. Make certain that you have your doctor's 24-hour phone number and the number of the maternity department at the hospital.

In most cases, your doctor will tell you to call her or report to the hospital when your contractions have been occurring about five minutes apart for at least one hour. If you have a history of very rapid labors, or if you live a long distance from the hospital, your doctor may advise you to come in earlier. Also, if your baby is in a breech position, if you are carrying twins, if you

have had a previous cesarean section, or if you have developed any other pregnancy complications, such as high blood pressure or diabetes, your doctor will probably instruct you to come to the hospital immediately if you think you are in labor.

If you ever experience contractions that you believe are labor and you are more than two weeks away from your due date, go to the hospital immediately. Premature labor can often be stopped with drugs, and this will avoid the delivery of a premature baby that may have difficulty surviving outside your body.

Also, if you feel a gush of fluid or even a slight leak coming from your vagina, go to the hospital immediately, even if you are not having labor contractions. These sensations may indicate that the

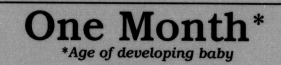

# One Month*
*Age of developing baby*

The letters within the black circles indicate the following organs and structures:

A Diaphragm
B Liver
C Stomach
D Pancreas
E Large intestine
F Abdominal muscle
G Small intestine
H Spinal cord
I Spine
J Uterus
K Bladder
L Cervix
M Rectum
N Pubic bone
O Urethra
P Clitoris
Q Labium
R Anus
S Vagina
T Fallopian tube
U Ovary
V Embryo

The numbered shadows surrounding the abdomen indicate the monthly growth of the abdomen. For example, the shadow labeled "3" indicates the size of the abdomen three months after conception.

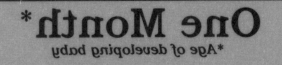

The letters within the black circles indicate the following organs and structures:

A Diaphragm
B Liver
C Stomach
D Pancreas
E Large intestine
F Abdominal muscle
G Small intestine
H Spinal cord
I Spine
J Uterus
K Bladder
L Cervix
M Rectum
N Pubic bone
O Urethra
P Clitoris
Q Labium
R Anus
S Vagina
T Fallopian tube
U Ovary
V Embryo

The numbered shadows surrounding the abdomen indicate the monthly growth of the abdomen. For example, the shadow labeled "3" indicates the size of the abdomen three months after conception.

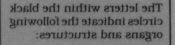

# Three Months*
*Age of developing baby

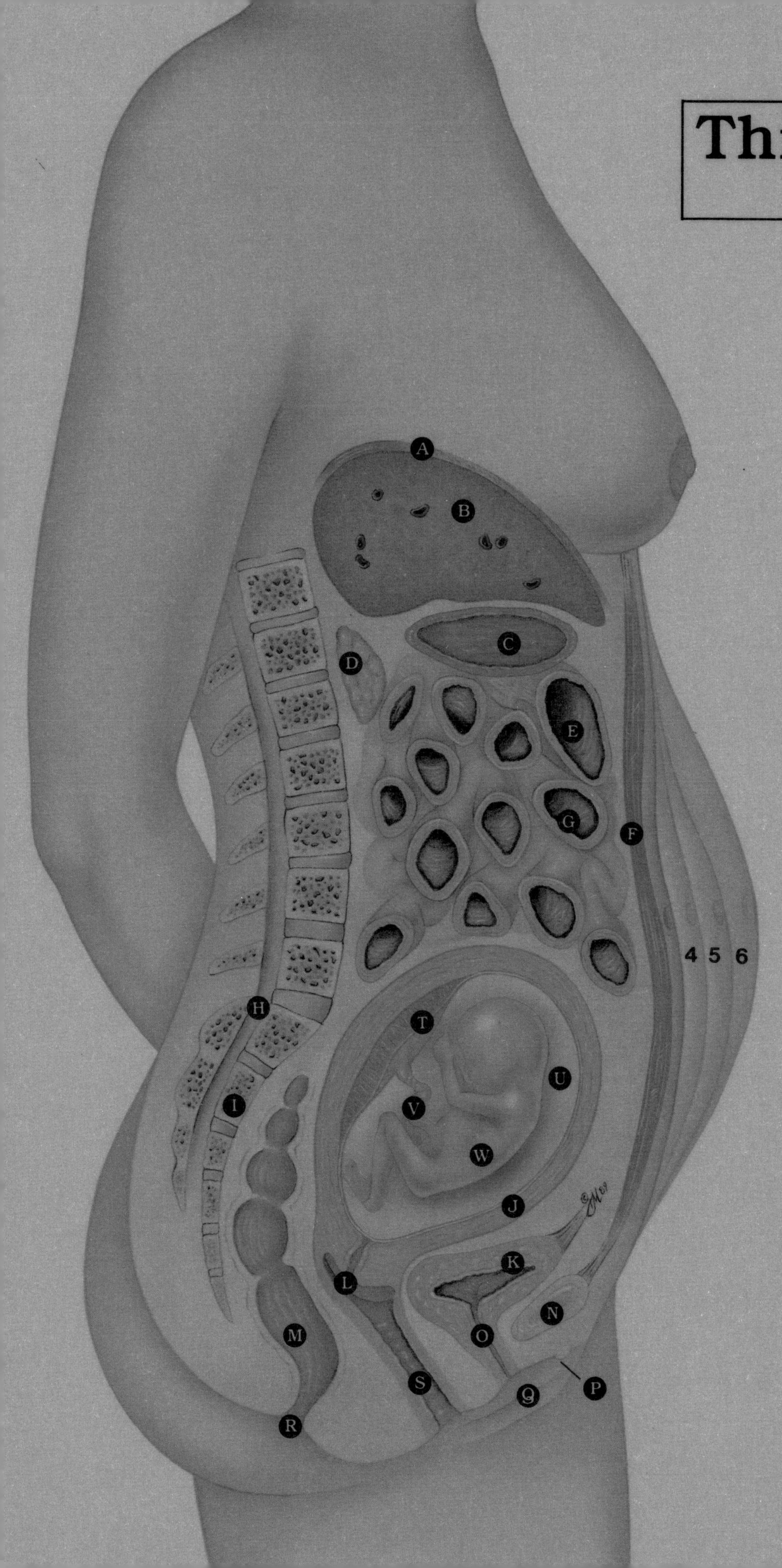

The letters within the black circles indicate the following organs and structures:

A Diaphragm
B Liver
C Stomach
D Pancreas
E Large intestine
F Abdominal muscle
G Small intestine
H Spinal cord
I Spine
J Uterus
K Bladder
L Cervix
M Rectum
N Pubic bone
O Urethra
P Clitoris
Q Labium
R Anus
S Vagina
T Placenta
U Amniotic sac
V Umbilical cord
W Fetus

The numbered shadows surrounding the abdomen indicate the monthly growth of the abdomen. For example, the shadow labeled "4" indicates the size of the abdomen four months after conception.

4 5 6

# Three Months*
*Age of developing baby

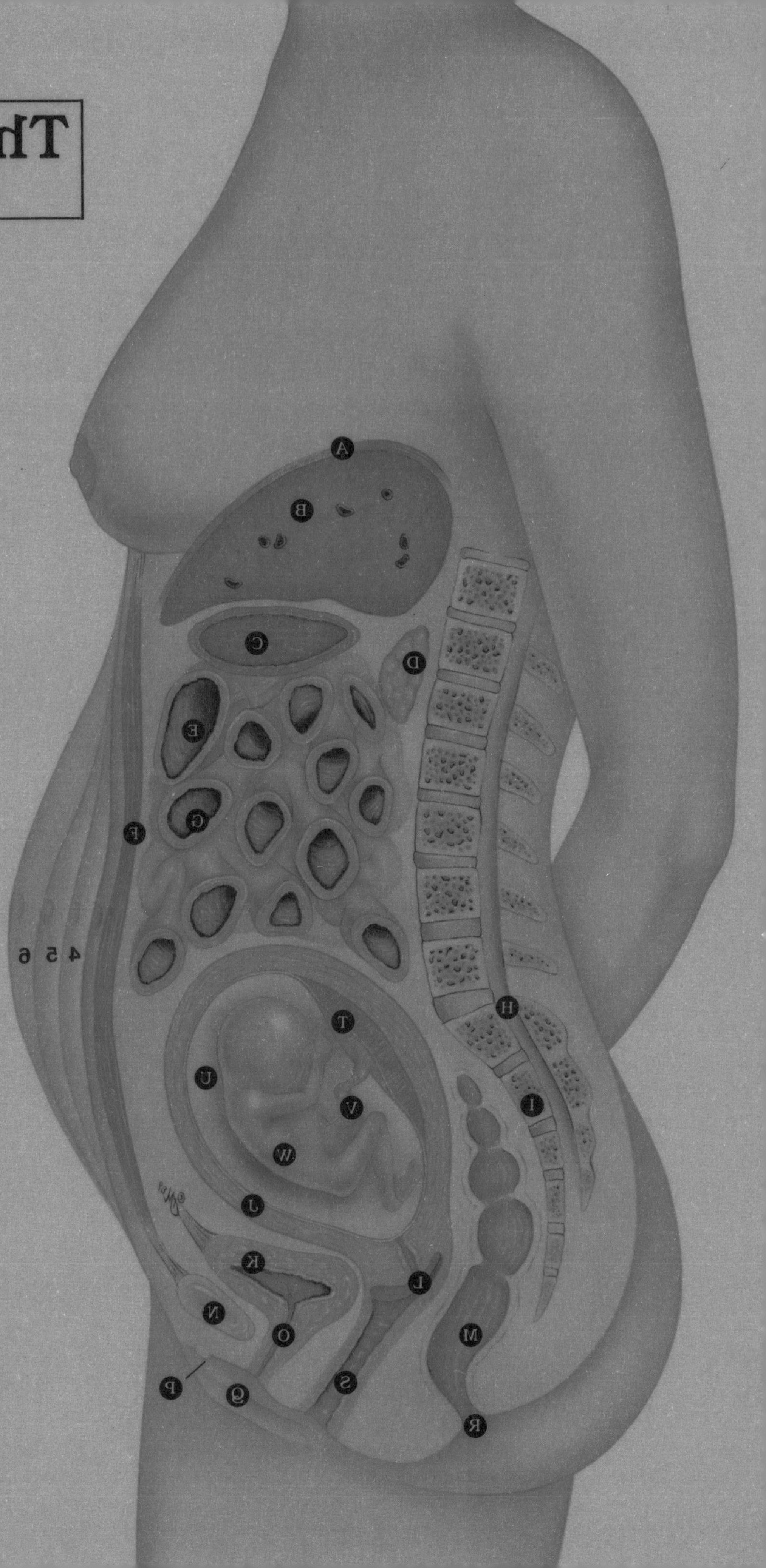

The letters within the black circles indicate the following organs and structures:

A Diaphragm
B Liver
C Stomach
D Pancreas
E Large intestine
F Abdominal muscle
G Small intestine
H Spinal cord
I Spine
J Uterus
K Bladder
L Cervix
M Rectum
N Pubic bone
O Urethra
P Clitoris
Q Labium
R Anus
S Vagina
T Placenta
U Amniotic sac
V Umbilical cord
W Fetus

The numbered shadows surrounding the abdomen indicate the monthly growth of the abdomen. For example, the shadow labeled "4" indicates the size of the abdomen four months after conception.

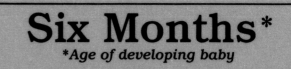

# Six Months*
### *Age of developing baby

The letters within the black circles indicate the following organs and structures:

A Diaphragm
B Liver
C Stomach
D Pancreas
E Large intestine
F Abdominal muscle
G Small intestine
H Spinal cord
I Spine
J Uterus
K Bladder
L Cervix
M Rectum
N Pubic bone
O Urethra
P Clitoris
Q Labium
R Anus
S Vagina
T Placenta
U Amniotic sac
V Umbilical cord
W Fetus

The numbered shadows surrounding the abdomen indicate the monthly growth of the abdomen. For example, the shadow labeled "7" indicates the size of the abdomen seven months after conception.

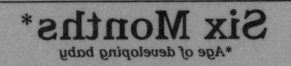

# Six Months*
## *Age of developing baby.

The letters within the black circles indicate the following organs and structures:

A Diaphragm
B Liver
C Stomach
D Pancreas
E Large intestine
F Abdominal muscle
G Small intestine
H Spinal cord
I Spine
J Uterus
K Bladder
L Cervix
M Rectum
N Pubic bone
O Urethra
P Clitoris
Q Labium
R Anus
S Vagina
T Placenta
U Amniotic sac
V Umbilical cord
W Fetus

The numbered shadows surrounding the abdomen indicate the monthly growth of the abdomen. For example, the shadow labeled "7" indicates the size of the abdomen seven months after conception.

# Nine Months*
("Lightening" has occurred)
*Age of developing baby

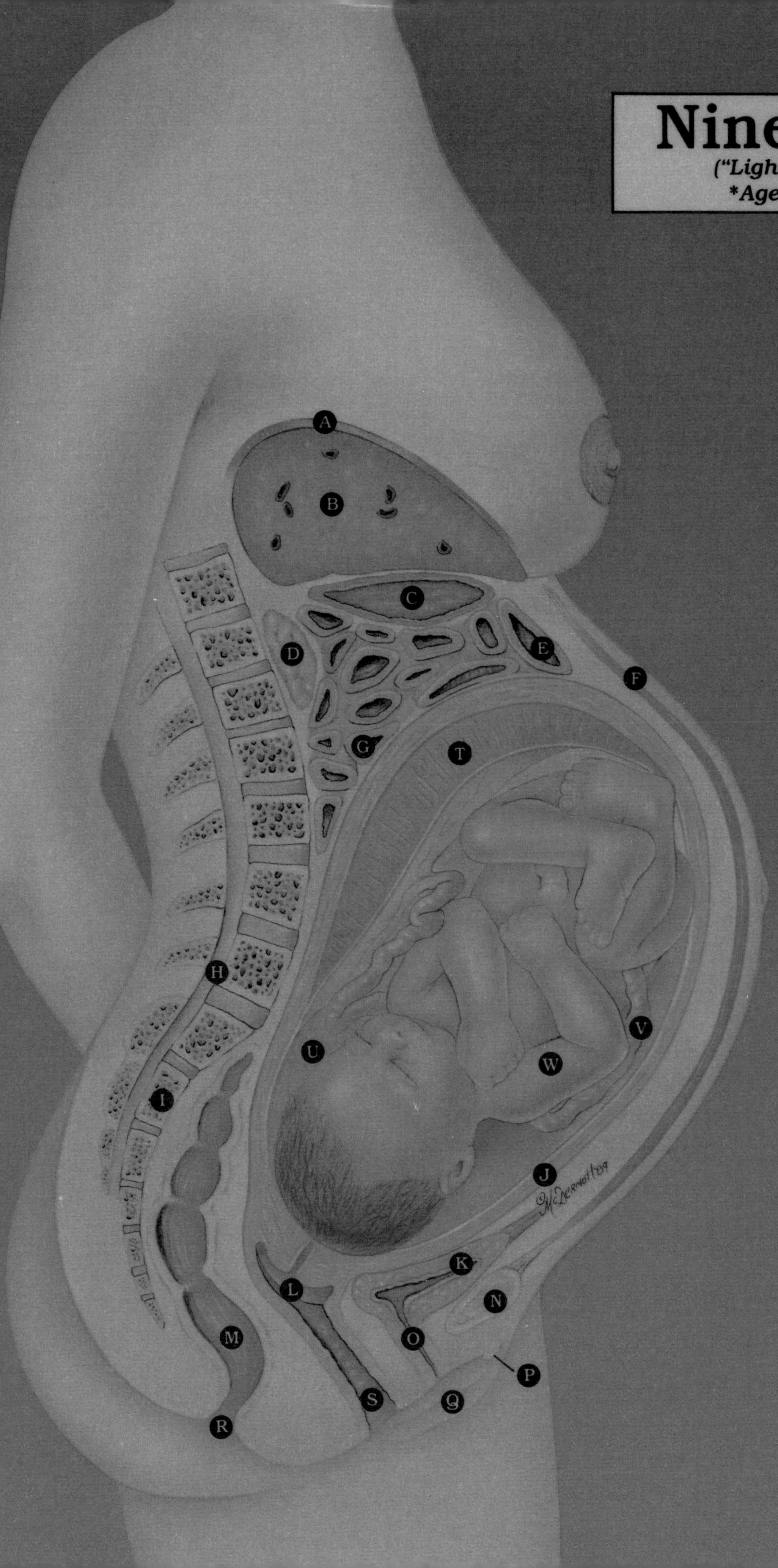

The letters within the black circles indicate the following organs and structures:

A Diaphragm
B Liver
C Stomach
D Pancreas
E Large intestine
F Abdominal muscle
G Small intestine
H Spinal cord
I Spine
J Uterus
K Bladder
L Cervix
M Rectum
N Pubic bone
O Urethra
P Clitoris
Q Labium
R Anus
S Vagina
T Placenta
U Amniotic sac
V Umbilical cord
W Fetus

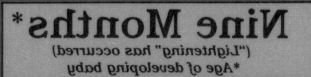

The letters within the black circles indicate the following organs and structures:

A Diaphragm
B Liver
C Stomach
D Pancreas
E Large intestine
F Abdominal muscle
G Small intestine
H Spinal cord
I Spine
J Uterus
K Bladder
L Cervix
M Rectum
N Pubic bone
O Urethra
P Clitoris
Q Labium
R Anus
S Vagina
T Placenta
U Amniotic sac
V Umbilical cord
W Fetus

amniotic sac, which forms a protective covering around the baby and keeps out harmful bacteria, may have ruptured.

Because of the uncertainty and discomfort that tend to occur during the first stage, it is a good idea to plan your method and route for getting to the hospital well before you actually go into labor. Can you reach your husband during the day if he is at work? Will road construction or rush-hour traffic cause you any delay? What are some alternate routes? Can a neighbor or friend take you to the hospital if you are unable to contact your husband? Make your plans well before labor begins so that you are not caught in a last-minute panic.

*Arrival at the hospital.* Upon your arrival at the hospital, your first stop may be the admitting office, where you will be asked to read and sign forms and indicate how you will pay for your hospital stay. Since hospital procedures vary considerably, it is a good idea to find out in advance about your hospital's admitting policies—especially the procedures for late-night and weekend admissions. Many hospitals will allow you to preregister so that you may avoid these procedures when you are going through the discomfort and the emotional ups and downs of the first stage of labor.

From the admitting office, you will go to the labor-and-delivery or maternity floor, where a doctor or nurse will greet you. A quick but thorough physical examination, including a vaginal examination to assess your degree of dilation and effacement, will be performed. The baby's heart rate, presentation, and position will also be checked. If you feel that you have ruptured your amniotic sac, a visual examination of the vagina may be performed to confirm this.

The type of routine care you will receive from this point on will vary widely from hospital to hospital. Feel free to discuss these proce-

dures with your doctor in advance and express your preferences. The following are common hospital procedures that may be performed.

*Enema in early labor.* An enema, which evacuates your rectum, may be performed to prevent stool from contaminating the vaginal area during the latter stages of labor and delivery. Some hospitals and doctors routinely prescribe an enema for all women during labor. Other hospitals and doctors consider it to be optional.

*Administration of intravenous fluids.* During labor, digestion stops, and any food or liquid in your stomach may cause you to vomit. For this reason, food is usually prohibited during labor, although small amounts of water or juices may be allowed. To prevent dehydration, intravenous fluids, commonly called "IVs," are usually given. To administer these fluids, the nurse or doctor will insert a small needle into a vein in your arm. The needle will then be attached to a length of plastic tubing, which will be connected to a bottle or a plastic bag filled with a sterile solution of water, sugar, and sodium (salt).

Hospitals and doctors also vary considerably on the routine administration of intravenous fluids, especially if the woman's labor is normal and no complications are expected. However, most doctors agree that intravenous fluids will be needed if the woman develops continuous nausea and vomiting, experiences a very long labor, or requires pain medication or anesthesia.

*Shaving of pubic hair.* In the past, it was customary to shave off all of a woman's pubic hair when she entered the hospital in labor. Today, this is no longer standard practice; many doctors believe that removal of the pubic hair is unnecessary. In some hospitals, a "mini-prep" is performed, in which only a small area of hair near the lower part of the vaginal opening is shaved.

*Restriction to bed.* Most hospitals will allow you to be out of bed—either walking, sitting, or squatting—during the early phases of labor. Once your uterine contractions become quite strong or you have been given pain medication, however, you should remain in bed for your own safety. If your blood pressure is abnormally high or if the baby's heart rate is abnormal, you should remain in bed for your entire labor.

*Vaginal examinations.* At regular intervals during your labor, usually every one to two hours, your doctor or nurse will examine your cervix by placing two gloved fingers into your vagina. This examination will be performed to determine the extent of effacement and dilation of the cervix. Such checks are usually kept to a minimum, however, to avoid introducing bacteria into the uterine cavity and causing infection.

*Electronic fetal monitoring.* One of the major advances in obstetrical care in the last two decades has been the ability to monitor the condition of the baby during labor. An electronic fetal monitor is an instrument that continuously records the baby's heart rate and the pattern of your uterine contractions. By looking at this recording, your doctor can determine not only the frequency, duration, and interval of your contractions, but also the well-being of your baby.

A fetal monitor may be used either externally or internally. In the external form of monitoring, two elastic belts are placed around your abdomen. On one belt is placed an ultrasound device to detect the baby's heartbeat, and on the other, a device to detect your contractions. In the internal form of monitoring, a small wire attached to the top of the baby's head detects the heartbeat, and a thin plastic tube inserted through your cervix and into the cavity of the uterus detects uterine contractions.

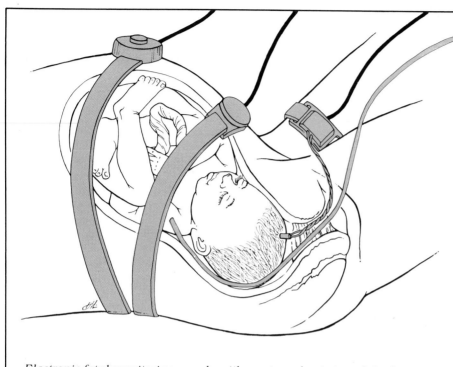

*Electronic fetal monitoring may be either external or internal. In the external form, two belts are placed on your abdomen, one holding a device to monitor the baby's heartbeat, the other holding a device to record your contractions. In the internal form, a small wire is attached to the baby's head to monitor his heartbeat and a plastic tube is inserted in your uterus to detect your contractions.*

Once settled in at the hospital, you will find a routine for handling contractions, perhaps based on what you learned in childbirth preparation classes. *Labor contractions should always be thought of as contractions and not as labor pains.* The following is a routine that many women learn and use successfully with their contractions.

1. Greet the contraction with a long sigh. As you breathe out, try to release all of your bodily tension.
2. At the same time, focus your attention in some way. For example, focus on your partner's face or a picture or object of your choice; close your eyes and "see" your cervix opening as your uterus contracts; picture yourself in a peaceful, relaxing place; focus on music of your choice, or the soothing sound of your husband's voice; or have your husband stroke you, and focus on the sensations.
3. Breathe slowly and easily.
4. Try to stay relaxed and limp through each contraction. It may help if you focus on one part of your body each time you exhale. Try to release tension in that part as you breathe out. Then focus on another part with the next breath.

You can follow this routine for each contraction and in any position that seems to make you more comfortable—lying down, sitting, standing, squatting, down on hands and knees. You can do this type of exercise in the car on the way to the hospital, in bed, in a chair, or in the hospital corridor.

These techniques and others are often effective in keeping pain within manageable limits for part or all of labor. Women who use them generally need less pain medication than women who don't. Indeed, some women do not use any pain medication when using these techniques. (Do not, however, get discouraged if you feel that you need pain medication; ask your nurse or doctor for it.)

The rate and pattern of the baby's heartbeat during labor has been found to accurately reflect how well he is receiving oxygen from the placenta. During the ninth month, the baby's heartbeat should remain within the range of 120 to 160 beats per minute. Any heart rate higher or lower than this may indicate that the baby is not receiving sufficient oxygen. An abnormal heart rate pattern during contractions may also indicate that the baby is not receiving enough oxygen.

Hospitals and doctors likewise vary in their views concerning the routine use of electronic fetal monitoring. Some believe that all women in labor should have electronic monitoring at all times. Others believe that electronic monitoring is not necessary for a woman experiencing a normal labor with no medical complications. However, electronic monitoring will be necessary if there is any doubt about the baby's condition.

***Mother's activity during the first stage of labor.*** During the first stage of labor, you may become serious and quiet, focused on only one thing—your labor. Jokes will not be funny, and world events will lose their importance. You will probably experience many emotional ups and downs in a relatively short period of time. You may feel discouraged and may cry from time to time, but if you accept labor as it comes and understand what is happening and what to expect, you will be able to recover from these down periods and go on. Support, encouragement, help, and comforting gestures from your partner, doctor, and nurse will be especially helpful at this time.

Some women learn several types, or levels, of breathing to use through different stages of labor. In addition to the slow method just described, some women use a lighter, faster, but still relaxing pattern. There are a variety of techniques, many of which you may learn in your childbirth preparation class.

Besides using a routine for each contraction, you should try to change your position every 20 or 30 minutes, go to the bathroom every hour or so, and sip liquids or suck on ice after every contraction. You will find these measures quite comforting.

You may also find that having hot packs placed on the lower portion of your abdomen, on your groin, and near your vagina and having cold packs placed on the lower part of your back will be very comforting. Having a cool, moist washcloth rubbed over your face and neck may also feel good. Being touched and rubbed, especially in tense, sore areas, such as the shoulders and lower part of the back, may help a great deal at this time. If you feel a bit out of control, it may help to have your husband hold you tightly or to have him hold your head gently but firmly in his hands.

Many women, especially first-time mothers, become extremely anxious about how rapidly their cervix is dilating. You, too, may ask "How can my cervix not be dilating when I am having such strong contractions?" Don't be discouraged if you are examined by your doctor and she tells you that your cervix is dilating slowly. More than likely, after your next examination, you will show a great deal of progress.

After your cervix has dilated to about seven to eight centimeters, you will usually find that your contractions become long, very strong, and more difficult to manage with your breathing and relaxation techniques. During this so-called "transition" phase, you

may feel almost out of control. This part of labor is the most difficult and the most physically and mentally demanding. You may actually feel that your body is running away with you, and that you are being swept along in a tide of intense sensations. Fortunately, this is the shortest phase of labor.

As your cervix dilates even more, you will feel an intense urge

---

## Pushing too soon may injure the cervix and may lead to heavy bleeding.

---

to push the baby out through your vagina. It will be very important for you to try to resist this urge if you are told that your cervix is not completely dilated. Pushing too soon may injure the cervix and vagina and may lead to heavy bleeding. Pushing before your cervix is ready may also cause it to swell and may slow down your progress.

It is also quite common during this phase to feel extremely nauseated; you may actually want to vomit. Hiccups may also occur, adding further to your discomfort. Another symptom typical during the transition period is trembling of your arms and legs; this can be a bit unnerving for your husband if he doesn't know what to expect. You may also feel extremely hot or extremely cold, and you may either throw off your blanket or feel the need for additional blankets.

During transition, it is also common to feel extremely irritable. You may not want to be touched at all. You may even scream at your husband and tell him to leave you alone. This is not uncommon, and he should understand that this

disagreeable mood will pass as the transition phase ends.

**The Second Stage.** Once your cervix has dilated to ten centimeters in diameter, the second stage of labor will begin. This is also called the "pushing" stage, since you will be directed to push with each contraction in order to force the baby down through your pelvis and vagina.

Your baby will actually be born during the second stage of labor. This stage ranges in length from 15 minutes to three hours or more. On average, if this is your first baby, the second stage will last about one hour; if you have had previous babies, it will last about 15 to 30 minutes.

When your cervix is completely dilated, the intense, out-of-control feelings will usually subside, and you will be ready to get down to the business of delivering your baby. The contractions often space out somewhat, and you may even get a short break from contractions (this is more likely with first-time mothers). It is always wonderful news when you are told that your cervix is completely dilated and you can begin pushing when you feel like it.

During the second stage, you may behave differently than in the first stage. You may find yourself holding your breath or slowly letting it out as you bear down (in a way that is similar to, but more intense than, what you do when you have a bowel movement). Relaxing the vaginal area as you bear down is especially important, because by tensing the muscles in this area, you will actually be fighting against the birth of your baby. It will also hurt much more if you tighten these muscles.

You will probably notice a real change in your contractions at this time. Most will contain a reflex need to strain or grunt, called an "urge to push," which will come and go about three to five times per contraction. With each urge to push, you will need to bear down.

Every time you bear down, you will push the baby closer to the outside world. It will be hard work and it will hurt, but it will also be an exciting time, with lots of cheering and praise for your efforts. Most women find that they have a new sense of energy and have the strength to keep pushing.

The best way to push is to push only when your body makes it happen—only when the urge to push comes. That way, you won't exhaust yourself, and you won't hold your breath so long that you or the baby get too little oxygen. The following is a routine many women use for pushing during second stage contractions.

1. Regardless of your position (reclining, lying on your side, squatting), greet the contraction with a long breath, and curl your body forward.
2. Breathe as you did during first stage contractions.
3. When you feel the reflex urge to push (it is unmistakable), follow it by grunting or holding your breath and bearing down. Make certain that as you are pushing, you are also consciously trying to relax your vaginal muscles. The urge to push will go away after a few seconds. When it does, breathe until the urge to push returns; then repeat this process through each urge until the contraction ends.
4. Relax or change position between contractions.

***Positions for the second stage.*** Unless the baby is coming fast, you will have time to change positions during the second stage. Many childbirth educators encourage women to learn to squat comfortably before labor because this is such a helpful position for the second stage. By squatting, you will be giving the baby more room to come down through your pelvis than he would have if you were in any other position. You will also be taking advantage of gravity in this position.

Lying on your side is a good position if the baby is coming fast, if you have painful hemorrhoids, or if you must lie down for some reason. Resting on your hands and knees may help if the baby is large or if his heartbeat has been slowing down during your contractions. Semi-sitting allows you to see your baby as he comes out. It is also a convenient position for your doctor.

***The birth of your baby.*** Once the top of the baby's head is visible at the opening of your vagina between contractions, your nurse will ready you for delivery. In some hospitals, you will be transferred to a specially equipped delivery room. If your hospital has an LDR room (labor-delivery-recovery room) or a birthing room, you will not be moved; rather, you will deliver your baby in the same bed in which you went through labor.

Once you are on the delivery table or labor bed, you will be asked to move your buttocks to the end of the table as you would during a routine pelvic examination in your doctor's office. Your legs will then be raised up and placed into either stirrups or leg platforms, unless you and your doctor have previously agreed that you will deliver without them. Once, all women gave birth lying on their back with their legs up in stirrups (the lithotomy position). Today, many doctors and midwives allow their patients to use other birth positions. You may, for example, be able to lie on your side with your upper leg raised and have your husband hold it up.

In whatever position you use, your thighs, vagina, and anal area will be washed with a warm antiseptic solution, and sterile drapes will be placed over your abdomen and thighs. Your husband may then be asked to sit on a stool by the head of your bed.

While preparations are being made for delivery, you will continue to have contractions and you will experience the urge to push. In some cases, your doctor may tell you to continue pushing. However,

if preparations are not complete, you may be asked to try not to push and instead to pant rapidly when you have the pushing urge.

After preparations for delivery are completed, you will be urged to push. You may ask if the head of the table or bed can be elevated to about a 35-degree angle so that you can push in a semi-upright position. This is usually much more effective than pushing when

> ## After preparations for delivery are completed, you will be urged to push.

you are flat on your back. Some hospitals may also have a wedge that can be placed under the mattress to achieve this position. Your partner can also help by holding up your shoulders as you push.

As you continue pushing, your baby will be making his way down through the pelvis and vagina; he will accommodate himself to their shape by turning his body and head. As the baby's head emerges, you will feel a great deal of stretching and burning in your vagina and pressure on your rectum. This will be an intense time. You'll know the baby is almost there, and you may be tempted to push as hard as you can to get him out quickly. That would be a mistake, however, because a sudden push could make the baby come out too quickly and tear your vagina and rectum. Your doctor will usually tell you when to stop pushing. Let your contractions do the work alone. You should pant rapidly and lightly, so that the baby will emerge gradually.

To prevent tearing of the vagina and rectum during delivery, your

## The Journey to Birth

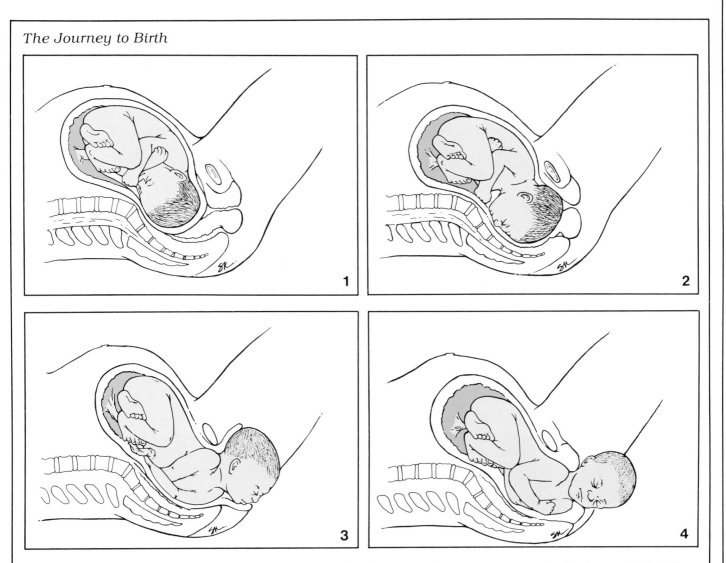

*Through the force of your contractions, your baby's head twists and turns to negotiate the birth canal. First, the baby's head bends forward to ease its way out of the uterus (1). Next, as the contractions continue, the baby's head is turned slightly and actually faces downward (2), so that the narrowest part of his head passes through your pelvis. Then his neck extends and his head is pressed upward and becomes visible through the vaginal opening (3). Once outside your body, his head is no longer guided by your contractions, and it once again becomes aligned with his shoulders (4). The rest of his body soon follows.*

doctor may perform an episiotomy. In this procedure, she will make a small incision through the skin and muscles from the lower portion of your vagina toward your anus. This will enlarge the opening of the vagina to allow for delivery of the baby's head. (The head is the largest part of the baby to come through your vagina.) If this is your first baby, you will probably need an episiotomy; if you have had previous babies, you will often not need an episiotomy since your vagina will have been stretched by previous deliveries.

The length and direction of the episiotomy will depend on the size of the baby's head and the elasticity of your vaginal tissues. In most cases, a midline episiotomy will be performed—straight down from the midpoint of the vaginal opening directly toward the anus. If the incision is made at an angle, it is called a mediolateral episiotomy. After the baby and placenta have been delivered, your doctor will sew the skin and muscles back together using sutures. The sutures will not have to be removed; they will dissolve on their own in about two weeks. You will, of course, be given

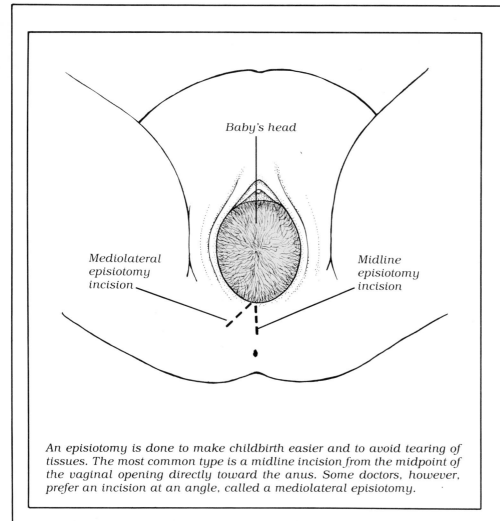

Baby's head

Mediolateral
episiotomy
incision

Midline
episiotomy
incision

*An episiotomy is done to make childbirth easier and to avoid tearing of tissues. The most common type is a midline incision from the midpoint of the vaginal opening directly toward the anus. Some doctors, however, prefer an incision at an angle, called a mediolateral episiotomy.*

a local anesthetic before the episiotomy is performed (unless the area is already numb from previous anesthesia), so that you will feel neither the incision nor the sewing. Not all doctors routinely perform episiotomies, so during your prenatal visits, ask your doctor if she thinks you will need to have one.

As the baby's head is delivered, your doctor may ask you to stop pushing, so that she may use a suction bulb to remove mucus from the baby's mouth and nose. As you again begin pushing, the upper shoulder, the lower shoulder, and then the rest of your baby will emerge. And what a sense of relief you will feel.

Your baby will usually begin crying on his own. (The doctor slapping an upside-down baby happens only in the movies). The doctor may then place the baby on a sterile sheet on your abdomen so that you may see and touch him. Next, the doctor will clamp the umbilical cord in two places and cut between the clamps. Since there are no nerves in the umbilical cord, neither you nor your baby will feel anything.

Once you have had a chance to hold your baby, he will probably be placed in a heated bassinet and carefully examined. His footprints will be taken and then he will be brought to your side.

**The Third Stage.** Your job will not end with the delivery of your baby. The placenta will need to be expelled. This third stage usually lasts from about five to thirty minutes. The nurse or doctor will keep a hand on your abdomen to determine when the placenta separates from the wall of your uterus. Then you will be asked to push it out. You may feel some cramping, but there is usually only slight discomfort. Your doctor will then carefully examine the placenta to make certain that no parts have been left inside your uterus to cause bleeding or infection.

**The Fourth Stage.** Immediately after birth, while you are admiring your new baby, your doctor will focus on your well-being. The condition of your uterus and vagina will be of major concern. It is important that your uterus remain contracted after birth to keep it from bleeding. Most women lose about one cup of blood at the time of birth. While this may seem like a lot, remember that among the many other changes of pregnancy, your blood supply greatly increases. Your doctor will watch the amount of blood lost immediately after birth and, if necessary, take measures to reduce the blood loss. These may include massaging your uterus vigorously or giving you an injection of a medication that will cause your uterus to contract.

Your doctor will also carefully examine your vagina and cervix to make certain there were no tears made during delivery. Although the idea of tearing sounds rather unpleasant, these tears are usually not serious and will heal rapidly.

For about the next two hours, you will remain in bed and your nurse will continue to check your recovery from labor and delivery. About every 15 minutes, she will check your pulse, blood pressure, and breathing rate. She will also check your vagina to make sure that you are not experiencing excessive bleeding.

## VARIATIONS OF NORMAL LABOR

The pattern of labor and delivery that has been described to this point is considered "normal," and chances are that this will be the course of your labor and delivery. However, some women may experience a deviation from this normal pattern. A woman's delivery may deviate for a variety of reasons, including the large size or unusual position of her baby, the small or abnormal size or shape of her pelvis, or the extended duration of her labor. If a problem should arise, your doctor will know the best course to follow. However, to be prepared for any deviation from the norm, you should understand the need for the following procedures.

**Forceps Delivery.** Forceps are spoon-shaped metal instruments (they've been compared to salad tongs in appearance) used to help in delivering the baby's head. If the force of your uterine contractions and your pushing efforts are not enough to deliver the baby, and if your second stage becomes excessively long (over two hours), your doctor may deliver the baby with forceps. Forceps may also be used if the baby's heartbeat slows rapidly during the second stage and an immediate delivery is necessary for the baby's health.

The doctor will insert the two separate blades of the forceps into your vagina on the sides of the baby's head. As you push, the doctor will pull gently on the handles of the forceps to deliver the baby's head. Sometimes forceps will leave small bruises on the baby's face. These marks are temporary and usually fade completely in about one week.

**Artificial Rupture of the Membranes.** Normally, during labor, or sometimes before labor, the membranes of the amniotic sac will rupture, releasing the amniotic fluid into your vagina. In some cases, your doctor may wish to artificially rupture the membranes by inserting a small plastic hook through your cervix and making a small hole in the membranes. This procedure often speeds up a slow labor. There will be no pain for you

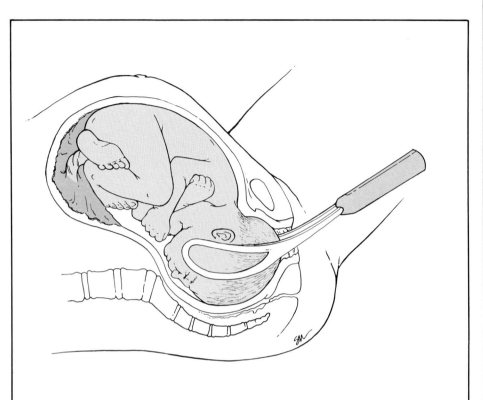

*Forceps may be used to help deliver the baby's head. The blades are slipped into your vagina and placed snugly on the sides of the baby's head. Then, as you push, the doctor will gently pull on the handles to ease the baby's head out.*

or your baby during this procedure, only the minor discomfort of a vaginal examination.

**Induction or Stimulation of Labor.** In some cases, your doctor may decide that it is time for the baby to be born, even though your labor contractions have not yet started. Your doctor may then induce labor. This is usually performed by giving you a hormone, called oxytocin, intravenously in the hospital. The labor contractions that are produced are usually similar to those that you would have during a normal labor, but they may be stronger in the beginning.

There are various reasons for inducing labor, including:

• The baby is overdue—that is, two weeks or more past the due date

• Health problems in the baby require immediate delivery
• The mother has certain medical problems, such as high blood pressure or diabetes, that can best be treated if the baby is delivered

Labor is never induced just because the parents think that a certain day would be convenient.

There are also certain circumstances when your doctor may need to stimulate or speed up contractions that have already begun. If you are having an unusually slow labor and the doctor has determined that the baby can safely pass through your pelvis, oxytocin can also be administered intravenously to make your contractions more intense and closer together.

**Cesarean Section.** Nearly 20 percent of deliveries in the United

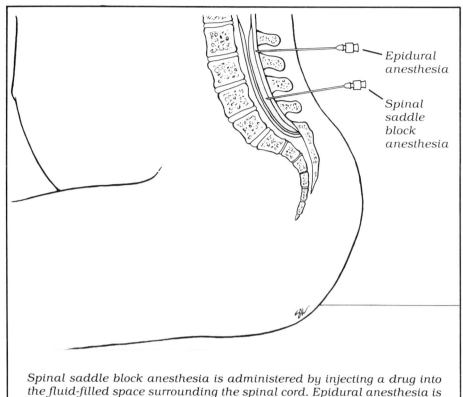

*Spinal saddle block anesthesia is administered by injecting a drug into the fluid-filled space surrounding the spinal cord. Epidural anesthesia is administered by injecting a drug into a space outside the covering of the spinal cord.*

States today occur by cesarean section. Recent medical advances have made this procedure much safer than it was a few decades ago. Cesarean section is performed in cases where a vaginal delivery would be hazardous for the baby, the mother, or both. A complete discussion of cesarean section can be found on page 100.

The preparation for a cesarean section will involve shaving the hair from your abdomen and then scrubbing the skin with an antiseptic solution. A thin, hollow rubber tube, called a catheter, will then be inserted into your bladder to drain off the urine. There will be many more people in the operating room than for a normal delivery, and each will have an important job to perform. These will include your doctor and an assistant, who will perform the surgery; at least two nurses, who will prepare surgical instruments for the doctor; the doctor who will administer the anesthesia; and the pediatrician, who will take care of the baby once it is delivered.

Depending upon your doctor's preferences and the condition of you and your baby, you will either be rendered unconscious by inhaling a gas (general anesthesia) or you will remain awake and will be given either a spinal or an epidural anesthetic (see *Ask the Doctor*, page 91) to numb the area from your navel to your toes. The spinal and epidural are both administered by injecting an anesthetic into an area in the lower spine. The entire operation will take about 30 to 90 minutes. After it is over, you will be moved to a recovery room where you will stay for about two to three hours, while a nurse carefully monitors your recovery. Since you will have had a major surgical procedure, you should expect to spend about four to seven days recovering in the hospital (this is only a few days longer than if you had a vaginal delivery).

Most couples have in their minds a clear expectation of how labor and delivery will occur for them. But it is important to remember that each labor and delivery experience is unique, and there may be times when this process does not go as smoothly as you may wish. Some couples feel guilty and blame themselves if cesarean section or a forceps delivery is required, thinking "If we had only done something different." For the most part, this is not so, since no one can know ahead of time exactly what will happen.

As your labor begins, accept it as uniquely yours, and understand that whatever procedures are performed are done for your health and the health of your baby. Remember, too, that no matter how smooth or how difficult your pregnancy, labor, and delivery are, they will fade to memories the moment you hold your beautiful new baby in your arms.

# Glossary

**Afterbirth:** Refers to the placenta and other specialized tissues associated with fetal development that are expelled after the delivery of the baby.

**Alpha-fetoprotein:** A substance formed in the fetus and excreted into the amniotic fluid. High levels of this substance in the mother's blood may indicate that the fetus has spina bifida or anencephaly. A test to detect this substance in the mother's blood is now generally performed on all pregnant women.

**Amniocentesis:** A prenatal diagnostic technique in which a needle is inserted through the mother's abdominal wall and into the uterus in order to remove a sample of amniotic fluid. The fluid is then analyzed to determine if certain abnormalities are present in the fetus.

**Amniotic fluid:** The liquid that fills the amniotic sac and surrounds and protects the developing fetus. The fluid usually contains cells shed by the fetus.

**Amniotic sac:** The bag in which the fetus and amniotic fluid are contained during pregnancy. Also called the "bag of waters."

**Analgesic:** A drug that inhibits the perception of pain.

**Anemia:** A condition in which the number or volume of red blood cells in the blood is abnormally low. Red blood cells are the oxygen-carrying component of blood.

**Anencephaly:** Failure of the brain to develop in the fetus.

**Anesthesia:** The loss of sensation that is medically induced to permit a painless surgical procedure. General anesthesia involves the entire body and produces loss of consciousness; regional and local anesthesia involve loss of sensation only in specific parts of the body.

**Anesthesiologist:** A doctor who specializes in the administration of anesthesia.

**Antibody:** A special kind of protein that is produced by the body's immune system to counteract or destroy foreign substances.

**Areola (*plural*, areolae):** The pink or brown circular area of skin that surrounds the nipple of the breast.

**Birth canal:** Vagina.

**Bloody show:** Blood-tinged mucus that is released from the cervix before or during labor.

**Braxton Hicks contractions:** Contractions of the uterus that occur before labor. Generally, they begin during the first trimester of pregnancy and occur irregularly until labor. They are felt as a tightening in the abdominal area.

**Breech presentation:** A fetal position in which the baby's feet or buttocks are nearest the cervix. *Compare to* cephalic presentation.

**Caudal anesthesia:** A form of regional anesthesia used for vaginal deliveries. It is achieved by injecting an anesthetic into an area of the lower spinal column.

**Cephalic presentation:** A fetal position in which the baby's head is nearest to the cervix.

**Cervix:** The lower portion of the uterus that opens into the vagina.

**Cesarean section:** Delivery of a baby through a cut made in the abdominal and uterine walls of the mother; used when the usual vaginal delivery is inadvisable or impossible.

**Chloasma:** A patchy, brownish discoloration of the skin of the mother's face during pregnancy.

**Chromosomes:** The structures within each cell that contain the genes.

**Colostrum:** The yellowish nourishing liquid secreted by the breasts shortly before and for a few days after childbirth until milk production begins.

**Dehydration:** Excessive loss of water from the body.

**Diabetes:** A disease in which the body cannot properly utilize carbohydrates because of insufficient production of insulin by the pancreas. While diabetes is generally chronic, there is a form of the disease, called gestational diabetes, that develops only during pregnancy and usually subsides after delivery. A woman who develops gestational diabetes, however, is more likely to develop chronic diabetes later in life.

**Diaphragm:** The muscle between the abdominal and chest cavities that is used in breathing.

**Diastasis recti:** Separation of the muscles in the middle of the abdomen.

**Dilation:** The enlarging of the cervical opening during labor, measured in centimeters.

**Doppler:** An instrument used to listen to faint sounds within the body; often used to detect the fetal heartbeat.

**Down's syndrome:** A birth defect in which a baby is born with an abnormal number of chromosomes. The disorder is marked by mental retardation and physical abnormalities.

**Eclampsia:** A serious and potentially fatal complication in pregnancy in which the pregnant woman develops high blood pressure, seizures (convulsions), and edema and has protein in her urine. *Compare* preeclampsia.

**Ectopic pregnancy:** A pregnancy in which the fertilized egg implants and begins to develop outside the uterus, usually in the fallopian tube but also in the ovary, on the cervix, or attached to another organ in the abdominal cavity.

**Edema:** Excessive accumulation of fluid; swelling.

**Effacement:** Softening, thinning, and shortening of the cervix that normally takes place just before or during labor.

**Embryo:** In humans, the developing baby from the time that the fertilized egg implants in the uterine wall until eight weeks after conception.

**Epidural:** A form of regional anesthesia used in both vaginal and cesarean deliveries. It is administered by injecting an anesthetic into a space outside the covering of the spinal cord.

**Episiotomy:** An incision made in the tissues around the vagina during the second stage of labor to make delivery of the baby's head easier and to avoid extensive tearing of the tissues.

**Estrogen:** A hormone produced by the ovaries and the placenta during pregnancy.

**Fallopian tube:** One of two tubes, which extend from the sides of the uterus, through which an egg passes after it is released from the ovary.

**False labor:** Irregular contractions of the uterus that do not result in dilation of the uterus.

**Fetal alcohol syndrome:** A condition that may develop in the developing baby of a mother who drinks alcohol during pregnancy; associated with physical abnormalities and mental retardation in the baby.

**Fetal monitor:** An electronic device used to record the baby's heart rate and the mother's uterine contractions during labor; may be used either internally or externally.

**Fetus:** A developing human from the eighth week after conception until birth.

**Fontanel:** A soft, membrane-covered space on a baby's head where skull bone has not yet grown; allows for easier passage of the baby's head through the vaginal canal during delivery.

**Forceps:** An instrument used to facilitate delivery of the baby's head.

**Fraternal twins:** Two babies that result from the fertilization of two separate eggs but that are carried in the uterus at the same time. They may or may not be of the same sex and generally have no more in common physically than do siblings resulting from separate pregnancies.

**Fundus:** The top portion of the uterus.

**Gestational diabetes:** *See* diabetes.

**Hemorrhoids:** Enlarged, blood-filled veins in the rectum.

**Herpes:** A recurring viral infection of the skin and mucous membranes. Painful blisters may occur around the mouth and sexual organs. It may be transmitted through direct contact with a sore, sexual contact, or from mother to baby during vaginal delivery.

**Hormone:** A chemical secreted in one part of the body and transported to another, where it regulates certain vital functions.

**Human chorionic gonadotropin:** A hormone produced by the placenta that stimulates the ovaries to produce estrogen and progesterone.

**Hypertension:** Abnormally high blood pressure.

**Identical twins:** Two babies that result from the fertilization of one egg and that are carried in the uterus at the same time; they are exactly alike in all physical traits.

**Infertility:** The inability to become pregnant.

**Labia (*singular,* labium):** the folds of skin and tissue at the opening of the vagina.

**Labor:** Progressive contractions of the uterus that lead to effacement and dilation of the uterus and the descent of the baby through the pelvic and vaginal canals.

**Lanugo hair:** The fine hair on the body of the fetus; it is sometimes present on the forehead, shoulders, and back of a newborn infant, especially one that was born prematurely.

**Lightening:** The descent of the baby into the pelvis; may occur before or during labor.

**Linea nigra:** A dark line that develops on the skin in the middle of the abdomen of a pregnant woman.

**Miscarriage:** Spontaneous expulsion of an embryo or of a fetus before it is capable of living outside the uterus.

**Mucous plug:** An accumulation of mucus in the cervical canal that serves to seal off the uterus during pregnancy.

**Ovulation:** The release of an egg from the ovary.

**Oxytocin:** A hormone secreted by the pituitary gland during labor to stimulate uterine contractions and milk secretion. A synthetic form is sometimes administered to initiate or speed up labor.

**Pelvis:** The bony structure in the mother through which the baby must pass during a vaginal delivery.

**Placenta:** The structure that develops within the uterus during pregnancy through which the fetus receives nourishment and oxygen and eliminates waste products; it also produces hormones that regulate changes in the mother's body during pregnancy and childbirth.

**Placental abruption:** Premature separation of the placenta from the uterine wall.

**Placenta previa:** A condition in which the placenta partially or completely covers the cervix, often causing vaginal bleeding before or during labor.

**Position:** The way the fetus is facing in relation to the mother's back.

**Preeclampsia:** A disorder of pregnancy, characterized by elevated blood pressure, edema, and kidney malfunction, that may precede the development of eclampsia.

**Premature:** Refers to birth that occurs before the thirty-seventh week of pregnancy.

**Presentation:** The position of the head of the fetus in relation to the cervix.

**Progesterone:** A hormone produced by the ovaries and placenta.

**Quickening:** The first fetal movements felt by the mother, usually occurring between the sixteenth and twentieth weeks after the last menstrual period.

**Rh factor:** A group of substances in the blood that stimulate the production of antibodies. Persons who have the Rh factor are termed Rh positive; those who lack it are called Rh negative.

**Rh incompatibility:** A condition in which an Rh-negative mother who has developed antibodies to the Rh factor becomes pregnant with an Rh-positive baby; this condition can lead to a form of anemia in the baby.

**RhO (D) immune globulin:** A substance injected into an Rh-negative woman shortly after she delivers an Rh-positive baby that destroys any Rh-positive blood cells that may have entered her body, thus preventing the development of antibodies against Rh-positive blood.

**Rubella:** A highly contagious viral infection, characterized by fever, a widespread pink rash, and enlargement of the lymph nodes in the neck. Although generally a minor disease, it can cause serious side effects in the fetus if contracted by a woman during pregnancy.

**Spider nevi:** Minute broken blood vessels that appear under the skin; spider veins.

**Spina bifida:** Failure of the spinal column to close completely in the fetus.

**Spinal anesthesia:** A form of regional anesthesia used in vaginal and cesarean deliveries; administered by injecting an anesthetic into the fluid-filled canal surrounding the spinal cord. *Compare to* epidural, caudal anesthesia.

**Stillbirth:** Delivery of a dead baby after the twenty-eighth week after conception.

**Stretch marks:** Streaks that develop on the abdomen, breasts, and thighs of a pregnant woman due to stretching of the skin; striae.

**Surfactant:** A substance produced by the fetal lungs that prevents them from collapsing at birth.

**Sutures:** Long, thin spaces between the bones of the developing baby's skull that allow the bones to slide over one another during delivery.

**Syphilis:** An infectious venereal disease that may be transmitted through sexual contact or from mother to baby.

**Tay-Sachs disease:** A fatal hereditary disease that affects the nervous system of the baby.

**Toxemia of pregnancy:** A serious disorder of pregnancy (encompassing preeclampsia and eclampsia) characterized by high blood pressure, edema, and kidney malfunction in the pregnant woman.

**Toxoplasmosis:** A disease that is transmitted either through contact with the feces of infected animals (especially cats) or through the consumption of undercooked, infected meat. Infection of a pregnant woman can cause fetal death or birth defects, especially mental retardation and blindness.

**Transition:** The period in the first stage of labor during which the cervix dilates from seven centimeters to ten centimeters.

**Transverse presentation:** A fetal position in which the fetus is lying perpendicular to the mother's body (i.e. sideways). Usually, the shoulder of the fetus is closest to the cervix.

**Trimester:** One of the three traditional divisions of pregnancy, each lasting approximately three months.

**Ultrasound:** Use of high-frequency sound waves to locate and produce an image of the fetus and placenta.

**Umbilical cord:** The structure through which fetal blood flows to and from the placenta to obtain oxygen and nutrients and eliminate fetal waste.

**Uterus:** The hollow, muscular organ of the female in which the fertilized egg implants and develops; womb.

**Vagina:** The six- to seven-inch-long muscular canal extending from the vulva to the uterus.

**Varicose veins:** Swollen, distended veins, usually in the legs.

**Vernix caseosa:** A protective, cheeselike substance that covers the skin of the fetus; some may be present in skin folds at birth.

**Vulva:** The external female genital organs surrounding the openings of the vagina and urethra.

# Index

## U

ultrasonography, 48–49
  and baby's age, 49
  and birth defects, 49
  and multiple births, 106
umbilical cord, 10, 37, 80
urinary tract infection, 58
urination, 11, 26–27, 47, 99
  and burning, 58
  and pain, 58
uterus, 10, 14, 108
  growth of, 23, 47
  during labor, 108–110
  lining of, 11

## V

vagina, 35, 89, 95
vaginal bleeding, 11, 12, 58
vaginal discharge, 11, 28, 35, 99
  as prelabor symptom, 82, 99
vaginal examination
  after delivery, 118
  at first prenatal visit, 14
  during labor, 108, 113
vaginal infection, 28, 35

varicose veins, 81, 92–93
vegetarian diet, 18
vernix caseosa, 68, 98
vision changes, 95
vitamins, 17, 20–21
vomiting. *See* morning sickness

## W

walking, 50, 52
warning signs, 58–59, 99
water pills, 66
weight gain, 16, 19, 24–25, 37
  and multiple births, 106
    rapid, 25, 76
weight loss during pregnancy, 19, 25
"wives' tales," 36–37
working, 38–41

## X

X rays, 32, 38–39

## Y

yolk sac, 10, 46